Volunteer Involvement

Jurgen Grotz · Ruth Leonard

Volunteer Involvement

An Introduction to Theory and Practice

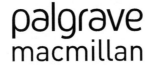

Jurgen Grotz
Institute for Volunteering Research
University of East Anglia
Norwich, UK

Ruth Leonard
Association of Volunteer Managers
London, UK

ISBN 978-3-031-19220-3   ISBN 978-3-031-19221-0   (eBook)
https://doi.org/10.1007/978-3-031-19221-0

This Palgrave Macmillan imprint is published by the registered company Springer Nature Switzerland AG
The registered company address is: Gewerbestrasse 11, 6330 Cham, Switzerland

We dedicate this book to all those who choose to be part of volunteer involvement, who continue to question what they see and themselves.

"Time is life itself, and life resides in the human heart." (Michael Ende)

Preface

The theory of volunteer involvement is built on accepting and understanding its complexity, recognising plurality and diversity. The practice of volunteer involvement requires responding to this complexity by creating volunteering relationships and making them succeed, continuously reflecting on context and change. The purpose of an introduction to the theory and practice of volunteer involvement is, in the words of the Vision of the Institute for Volunteering Research (2022), to:

> *"…bring about a world in which the power and energy of volunteering and the difference volunteering and volunteering research make to individuals and communities is well understood, so that individuals can be confident and feel safe about their decision to volunteer and communities grow stronger".*

And in the words of the Association of Volunteer Managers (2022) as part of:

> *"… connecting leaders of volunteering to make change happen together"* and to *"…inspire and empower leaders of volunteering".*

The idea for this book was first raised after a particularly pleasant lunch, in October 2019 when we, the two authors, were walking around the picturesque lake on the campus of the University of East Anglia. Without planning it, our meeting and discussion were grounded in a shared belief that some of the basic ingredients of volunteer involvement are conviviality, respect and enjoyment. As we talked, we also found that we shared the following fundamental views on volunteer involvement as:

- an example of our humanity,
- being conceived in many different ways,
- not an inherently good thing,
- based on relationships,
- needing both individual action and constant reflection.

We further shared with each other some of the many instances we had come across over the years, when organisations began to think of volunteer involvement as a good idea, but then commenced to plan as if they were intent on reinventing the wheel, not making use of any of the substantial existing knowledge. More recently, we have also received requests for information, such as from a college introducing a module on basic volunteer involvement or an umbrella organisation for a group of specialised and very small charities. We felt a basic introduction to theory and practice might be especially helpful in those circumstances.

We also agreed that the publicly observable conversations about volunteer involvement rarely seemed to reflect any of the five fundamental statements listed above, nor any serious reflections on key ingredients of volunteer involvement, such as 'choice'.

So, we decided to write this book to share some of our thinking around the basic ingredients and fundamental views on volunteer involvement. However, because we really didn't want to write yet another rulebook, we decided to offer a broad and balanced background picture of thinking about volunteer involvement, to encourage all those who want to involve volunteers and policymakers influencing volunteer involvement to think and act together, collaboratively and respectfully, and also to critically reflect on volunteer involvement.

And then along came a pandemic. Today, as we slowly and cautiously emerge from two years of personal and professional effects of the pandemic, it seems to us that even after the tremendous, shared experience of living, and volunteering, together through the pandemic, the conversations about volunteer involvement still appear broadly the same. Having said that, in England, possibly in response to the experiences during the pandemic, a new conversation has begun concerning a 'Vision for Volunteering' and we will seek to add our thinking to this.

Between us, we the two authors, have been involved as volunteers and with volunteers for several decades. From volunteering with young people in the YMCA and with disabled people, supporting sports for visually impaired people, to volunteering on telephone helplines, with Parent and Teachers Associations and as School Governor, to volunteering on a social activist newsletter, being a community mediator, as a peer mentor and to volunteering as trustees. We have also been involving volunteers in our roles as paid members of staff or as volunteers and we currently lead organisations that deal specifically with volunteering, both in research and practice.

When we started as volunteers, we could be involved in diverse activities. Many activities, especially those involving young people, were meant to be transformative. However, over our years of involvement, while activities have remained diverse, our conversations about volunteer involvement, in our professional roles, seem increasingly disconnected from that diversity. A much stronger single focus has developed on volunteering as 'service' or 'unpaid work'. Also, the activities of voluntary and community organisations, delivered by paid staff, are often unhelpfully conflated with volunteer involvement. This can blur the picture and can distort the conversation. Over the years of involvement, again and again, we had conversations regarding the many aspects of volunteering which were severely hampered by a lack of shared understanding of what we mean by volunteer involvement. And in England, since 2010, this was exacerbated by the absence of a shared vision for volunteering among those who involve volunteers, made worse as in some areas financial state support for volunteer involvement has all but disappeared.

We believe that it is important for all of us, who want to involve volunteers, to fully understand what volunteering encompasses and to critically reflect on our practice. We therefore want to offer, in one place, the broad background thinking about volunteering, hopefully supporting those who want to involve volunteers to hold balanced conversations and to reflect on practice. We come to this book with different backgrounds using different sources and language. We therefore deliberately chose to include a wide range of sources, seeking a language that is engaging and informative to practitioners, policymakers and funders as well as researchers. However, that makes this neither a solely academic nor a solely practitioner orientated book. We hope that this deliberate combination of knowledges, rather than depriving either, enriches both and supports inclusive conversations. By collaborating as practitioners and researchers, both with personal experience of volunteering and volunteer involvement, we approached this book in the way we will suggest to approach volunteer involvement.

And on the 100th anniversary of the publication of Ulysses by James Joyce, it seems fitting to recognise that Leopold Bloom, one of the main fictional protagonists in that novel, while wandering through Dublin thinks and acts to help others, doing so with kind curiosity. We too want to explore the theory and practice of volunteer involvement with kind curiosity. We reckon that not everybody will agree with everything in this book and we think that that's a good thing, but we hope that you too will consider what we put forward with kind curiosity.

This book is entitled 'Volunteer Involvement'. Those two words have been chosen carefully and deliberately, because there is much confusion relating to what volunteering is and what we should call it. Volunteers are involved in a huge variety of activities and operate in a diversity of organisational settings. From our point of view, there is no single model or approach to describe volunteer involvement. There are many models and approaches that emerge as volunteer involvement brings people together, connecting, collaborating, challenging and changing. We approach volunteer involvement as a concept including plurality, choice and personal responsibility. We respect that volunteer involvement reflects the ways in which volunteers, volunteer involving organisations, society and the state approach it and that the way they approach volunteer involvement reflects directly on personal and political ideologies, the society people wish to live in, and their attitudes to equality, diversity, inclusion, power and privilege. Volunteer involvement is, as this book recognises from the outset, diverse and contentious.

While writing this book, we talked to volunteers who told us that they had never really wondered what volunteering is and asked bluntly 'why do we need to know?' Our equally blunt answer is that for a positive volunteer experience, people do not need to know. They don't need to read this book and frankly, they might not want to either. Recognising this, we therefore must accept that this book is more for those who want to involve volunteers, rather than volunteers themselves. Nonetheless, we hope volunteers may be interested in some sections, or will come across them in inductions or training. We also hope that the content of this book is of relevance to those volunteers who involve other volunteers.

This book is therefore for those who want to think and learn about volunteer involvement and also to put their thinking and learning into practice, and to critically reflect on what they hear, what they see and what they plan. We think it can be useful for all who seek to involve volunteers, across the spectrum of volunteering, from those who:

- take part in self-organised associations without paid staff, like the Mutual Aid Groups established in England to respond to the COVID-19 emergency during the first March 2020 lockdown,
- volunteer in the tens of thousands of small, registered charities such as Parent-Teacher Associations, Sports Clubs and local Amateur Theatres,
- involve volunteers in large national charities and public services in areas including health, social care, education and conservation,
- develop and implement policies that influence volunteering, in local and national government, in the UK National Health Service, in universities and in private sector companies.

In this book, we encourage reflection rather than giving instructions. We offer a critical view of volunteer involvement, of where we have been, where we are, and want to get to, and we call on you, the reader, to join us in critical thinking. We expect people to use this book and its references alongside the numerous manuals, toolkits and instruction handbooks guiding specific areas of activity, like health and social care or criminal justice. However, this book will not just restate established advice but start from the premise that good practice in volunteer involvement, will not rest on prescribed, pre-defined instructions but on the need to be able to develop these for yourselves, through collaborating with others, putting your own thinking into practice. We think that volunteer involvement needs to be responsive to the specific circumstances of everyone affected. And, to make a lasting difference, it needs to be inclusive.

In the chapters that follow, we will lay out basic information on volunteering. At all stages, we will encourage you, the reader, to reflect on what we are saying, what others are saying, what you are thinking and how you put your thinking into practice. We have added 20 'Exercises' and nine 'Practice Examples' encouraging you to ponder what volunteering is and isn't and how it is undertaken, so encouraging you to reflect, not follow instructions. As volunteer involvement is such a large and complex topic, we have divided the book into six chapters. The first three broadly deal with theory and the remainder with practice.

In Chapter One, we discuss the complexity of volunteer involvement, in particular, what volunteering is and how we speak of it, reflecting our view that volunteer involvement stands as an example of our humanity and is not to be reduced to a single concept of unpaid labour. Chapter One is possibly a little mundane and maybe dull, especially when we present and discuss definitions, but it is necessary that we lay out clearly what terms we use, so that there isn't any misunderstanding in the subsequent chapters.

In Chapter Two, we consider the plurality of volunteer involvement concepts, in particular, how volunteering started, how people think about it and how this is constantly changing, reflecting that volunteer involvement can be conceptualised in many different ways and that those discussing it should take into account other knowledges and views. Chapter Two may contain much that seems familiar, but might not always be presented together in one place.

In Chapter Three, we explore volunteer involvement's diversity, in particular, we get to something that many colleagues don't seem to want to share. But we think it is now called for to seriously discuss negative views and impacts of volunteering, misconduct and the benefit fallacy, reflecting that volunteer involvement isn't an inherently good thing. Some of what you read or what we encourage you to reflect on in Chapter Three might be uncomfortable.

In Chapter Four, we get to relationships. We look at volunteer involvement in practice, like the connections volunteers make through volunteer involvement over time, reflecting that volunteer involvement is based entirely on relationships. We hope you can locate the volunteer involvement you are currently undertaking or are interested in and we will encourage you to apply some of your reflections from the first three chapters to your own practice.

In Chapter Five, we turn to reflection. We will use nine case studies to look in detail at issues that could arise during volunteer involvement reflecting that volunteer involvement will get better when we consider our practice in light of circumstances, rather than following general instructions.

Finally, in Chapter Six, we will consider how all this may relate to the future of volunteer involvement under the five core statements of the book, which together opened this Preface and separately each of the chapters. We hope that this will contribute to the upcoming conversations, not just concerning a 'Vision for Volunteering' in England, but more broadly on how we deal with the theory and practice of volunteer involvement.

Having fun yet? If all this sounds daunting, we will aim throughout to support you to find enjoyment in reading this book and in volunteer involvement. It may not often be said, but if volunteer involvement is not at least a little bit enjoyable, people will not do it for long. Volunteering is about relationships, with people being interested in coming together to make a difference, in often difficult circumstances. Those relationships will falter if they are not nurtured. Therefore conviviality, respect and enjoyment should always be basic ingredients of volunteer involvement and we strongly believe that kind curiosity should underpin how we approach the debate about it.

Norwich, UK   Jurgen Grotz
London, UK   Ruth Leonard

Acknowledgements

We wish to thank all the many volunteers, those who involve volunteers and make volunteer involvement happen as well as many other professionals and individuals whose activities and views have inspired us to write this book and keep us going.

We particularly want to thank Shaun Delaney, Claudia Demuth, Sally Dyson, Mike Locke, Fiona Poland, Melanie Price and Colin Rochester for their constructive comments on early drafts of this book.

Contents

About the Authors

Jurgen Grotz Ph.D. is Director of the Institute for Volunteering Research (IVR) at the University of East Anglia. He is Chair of the Association for Research in the Voluntary and Community Sector and trustee of the Voluntary Sector Studies Network. With three decades of experience in applied research, his largely interdisciplinary work has a strong focus on participative approaches and public engagement, working across the academic, public and voluntary and community sectors. He has co-edited the Palgrave Handbook of Volunteering, Civic Participation, and Nonprofit Associations (2016), is a co-author of Patient and Public Involvement in Health and Social Care Research: An Introduction to Theory and Practice (2020) and most recently co-edited Mobilising Voluntary Action in the UK—Learning from the Pandemic (2022).

Ruth Leonard is Chair of the UK's Association of Volunteer Managers whose day job is Head of Volunteering Development and Operations at Macmillan Cancer Support.

Ruth has been involved in volunteer management for over two decades and she has significant experience at providing leadership on involving and engaging people and is committed to ensure that others are able to develop these skills. She has written and spoken about volunteering for various publications and events, including chairing conferences on volunteer management and also safeguarding. Ruth is regularly asked to provide her practitioner's views and expertise to act as consultant for research on mobilising voluntary action.

Abbreviations

AVM	Association of Volunteer Managers
DBS	Disclosure and Barring Service
ESV	Employer Supported Volunteering
LSE	London School of Economic and Political Science
HR	Human Resources
IVR	Institute for Volunteering Research
NAVCA	National Association for Voluntary and Community Action
NCADC	National Coalition of Anti-Deportation Campaigns
NCS	National Citizen Service
NCVO	National Council for Voluntary Organisations
NHS	National Health Service
PSV	Police Support Volunteers
PVG	Protecting Vulnerable Groups Scheme
RSPB	Royal Society for the Protection of Birds
RNLI	Royal National Lifeboat Institution
TUC	Trades Union Congress
VCSE	Voluntary, Community and Social Enterprise
WCVA	Wales Council for Voluntary Action

List of Figures

List of Tables

1

Introduction

Abstract This chapter clarifies terminology and definitions, describes the places where volunteering takes place and discusses the complexity of volunteer involvement. It encourages the reader to use four 'Exercises' to reflect on what volunteering is, where it takes place, who should organise it and what the motivations of volunteers are.

Keywords Definitions · Theory · Concepts

Volunteer involvement stands as an example of our humanity. The impulse to do something which makes a difference to others, without being forced to do so, and without expecting financial or other direct, concrete rewards, can be found in people around the globe. It is something that can define us as being human. Much of volunteer involvement, possibly most, happens when neighbours, friends or even strangers come together in a common cause, but volunteer involvement also takes place through hundreds of thousands of organisations such as clubs and charities, many without and some with paid staff. In the UK, it is now

J. Grotz and R. Leonard, *Volunteer Involvement*,
https://doi.org/10.1007/978-3-031-19221-0_1

broadly acknowledged that volunteering takes place in all areas of society and that it makes a big difference to communities.

> …volunteering across communities helps bring people together, and makes them feel part of a greater whole by sharing with others from different backgrounds, helping those who have had a less than good start in life… (Commission on the Future of Volunteering, 2008, p. 3)

However, while volunteer involvement can be found everywhere in society, different individuals or groups see different meaning behind the words and there is no agreement regarding what the term 'volunteering' and the concept behind it encapsulate or how volunteer involvement should take place and why. When people got together to support others during the COVID-19 pandemic, some just wanted to help while others wanted to set up sustainable groups. Trustees of a charity, who are also volunteers, might seek to involve volunteers differently even within the same charity because they don't share a view on the purpose of volunteering within the organisation. The executive team of a large organisation involving volunteers may have a very different rationale for resourcing volunteer involvement compared to the teams of paid volunteer coordinators in their organisations, who directly involve volunteers. And in some contexts, like in the new Integrated Care Systems, people from National Health Service (NHS), local government, voluntary, community and social enterprise (VCSE) organisations and other partners come together with different knowledges and approaches to consider the role of volunteers in health and social care or in patient voice.

This means we want to begin this book by offering examples of different ways that words and concepts are interpreted and then be clear which terms and concepts will be used in this book and why. We will look at how to define volunteering, give examples of where and how people volunteer, look at the different organisations involving volunteers and at the end of the chapter provide estimates of how many people volunteer and why.

However, before we go on, we want to encourage you to consider your own thinking about volunteering. We suggest you do this by turning an important question on its head, by asking yourself how you would answer the following question in Exercise 1.1 finding your own examples of: 'What is definitely NOT volunteering?'

Exercise 1.1

What is definitely NOT volunteering? Why?

Excluding activities that are paid work, or that people are forced to do or that are for the benefit of one's family, think of examples that you would describe as definitely NOT being volunteering. For example, are any of the following definitely NOT volunteering:

- Is it volunteering to hold 'bed-ins for peace', like John Lennon and Yoko Ono did in 1969, as protest against wars?
- Is it volunteering to decorate your street with 'yarn bombing'?
- Is it volunteering to drive a bunch of kids to a football match, including your own?
- Is it volunteering for people to meet in 'men's sheds' to chat and maybe build something together?
- Is it volunteering to run a sponsored marathon?
- Is it volunteering to enter Government buildings en masse like the people who stormed the United States Capitol, 6th January 2021?
- Is it volunteering when tourists pay for activities and opportunities to assist abroad?
- Is it volunteering when people protest by gluing themselves to roads or railings?
- Is it volunteering to be a shop steward for a trade union?
- Is it volunteering to regularly get milk and bits and pieces for an ill neighbour?
- Is it volunteering to complete an online petition?
- Is it volunteering to organise a regular bridge evening?

1.1 What Is Volunteering?

There are no universally agreed terms and definitions for volunteering. In this section, we will explain why we use the term 'volunteering' and why we use the following definition:

> Volunteering is an individual's activity undertaken by choice, without concern for financial gain and intended to make a difference outside one's own family.

The above definition draws on the UK Volunteering Forum's 1998 definition (Cited in Kearney, 2001), using the core components of activities that are unpaid, uncoerced and making a difference. The above definition excludes terms such as 'benefit' and 'commitment' and does not identify specific areas of society in which the activity takes place. We don't use 'benefit' in the definition because people do not necessarily agree on what would be a benefit and the inclusion of 'benefit' may lead to a bias towards positive reporting (Grotz, 2011). We also don't use 'commitment' because it suggests the requirement of ongoing involvement. However, we continue to exclude activities solely directed at one's own family. As with other definitions, we exclude this to maintain a clear distinction between volunteering and caring obligations. The three core components as above and the exclusion of activities directed solely at one's own family appear in most common conceptualisations of volunteering in English in the UK, and have remained largely unchallenged over at least two decades. They have been widely used to define volunteering in academic literature since the end of the last millennium (Cnaan et al., 1996; Hustinx et al., 2010; Smith et al., 2016; Wilson, 2000). They also encapsulate what the United Nations described as volunteering in 2001a and still uses to describe it.

> ....the terms volunteering, volunteerism and voluntary activities refer to a wide range of activities, including traditional forms of mutual aid and self-help, formal service delivery and other forms of civic participation, undertaken of free will, for the **general public good** and where monetary reward is not the principal motivating factor. (United Nations General Assembly, 2001a, bold emphasis by the authors)

However, there are many definitions which add to or alter those core components. The United Nations wording above speaks of the 'general public good' and expands on the concept of unpaid. The UK Volunteering Forum's definition suggests that volunteering has to be 'for the benefit to society and the community'.

Volunteering is an activity that involves the "commitment of time and energy **for the benefit of society and the community** and can take many forms. It is undertaken freely and by choice, without concern for financial gain". (Kearney, 2001, p. 4, bold emphasis by the authors)

The UK Home Office, with powers on immigration, in May 2021 advised case workers assessing applications for asylum, as follows, defining where and how volunteering is taking place:

Volunteers are those who give their time for free **to charitable or public sector organisations** without any contractual obligation or entitlement. They are not employees or workers as defined by various statutory provisions. (Home Office, 2021, p. 18, bold emphasis by the authors)

The way these definitions are written depends on who writes them and for what purpose they are being used. Furthermore, these English language definitions do not accurately reflect the multiple and varying characteristics and culturally encoded concepts associated with volunteering captured in the UK alone, where over 200 languages are spoken, and where ideologies and individual backgrounds also affect how people think of volunteering.

Concepts of volunteering are further complicated by writers, practitioners and policymakers using different words with the same meaning, of what the term volunteering and its definition encapsulate. The United Nations don't just use the term 'volunteering' but also 'voluntary activity' and then locates a range of activities within this including 'mutual aid', 'service delivery' and 'civic participation'. The British economist and social reformer William Beveridge speaks of 'voluntary action' and describes it as broad-ranging, suggesting that "*The essence of Voluntary Activity is that it should not be stereotyped*" (Beveridge 1948, p. 12). Moreover, policymakers have tried at times to avoid the term volunteering and deliberately using alternatives such as 'social action', while continuing to use 'volunteering' interchangeably. A resource on enabling 'social action' from Department for Culture Media and Sport and the New Economics Foundation takes the following approach:

> Social action is about people coming together to help improve their lives and solve the problems that are important in their communities. It involves people giving their time and other resources for the common good, in a range of forms – from volunteering and community-owned services to community organising or simple neighbourly acts. (Department for Culture Media and Sport, n.d., p. 2)

There are also plenty of examples when people do not wish to identify themselves as volunteers but rather, as activists, campaigners or simply as someone who helps others. In this context, it is extremely easy, and unfortunately common, for people to use the same terms but mean different things or to mean the same thing and use different terms. Importantly, as we will explain in Chapter 3 what terms are used and how, are not just a question of choice but reflect personal and political ideologies. That is why we are encouraging not just carefully selecting terms and definitions but also recommending reflecting on the terms other people use and why.

Having explained the definition we use and why, we now explain why we use the word 'volunteering' to identify with its Latin core *voluntas*. In the English word 'voluntary', this focuses attention on volunteering reflecting an individual's will, intent, and determination, sometimes also referred to as agency. We think of volunteering as an individual's choice, deciding what to volunteer for and how, and what difference to make. The individual volunteer's choice shapes the community in which they want to live, and the power and resources to make that choice. In this book, the word 'volunteering' encapsulates the widest possible context, not restricted to particular areas. It captures activities that are undertaken through organisations and those that are not, as long as the activities reflect the three core components 'choice', 'not primarily for financial gain', 'making a difference' and the restriction of being 'outside one's own family' or at least not solely within and for one's own family. Thinking back to the examples in Exercise 1.1, all of them easily fit our definition.

Having explained our selection and definition of the term 'volunteering', we will next look at where volunteering happens. But first please consider the following question, about the most unusual places you can think of where volunteering takes place. See Exercise 1.2.

Exercise 1.2

Using the definition from this book

Volunteering is an individual's activity undertaken by choice, without concern for financial gain and intended to make a difference outside one's own family.

Try to think of the most unusual places you have heard of or can imagine, where activities take place that you would describe as definitely being volunteering.

- How about organising unusual activities such as:
  - the Tar Barrels Festival of Ottery St Mary in Devon,
  - the Cooper's Hill Cheese-Rolling and Wake near Gloucester,
  - or the World Stone Skimming Championships on Easdale Island in Scotland?
- How about counting birds in your garden or corals on a reef?
- How about visiting patients in hospital, singing for them?
- How about looking at photos of deep space online and marking any changes?

1.2 Where Does Volunteering Take Place?

It would be impossible to list in this book all examples of places where volunteering happens, so we will overview this by grouping examples. Five types are commonly used to categorise volunteering. In alphabetical order, they are: Campaigning, Mutual Aid, Leisure, Participation and Service (United Nations Volunteers Programme, 2021). Perhaps confusingly, each of these categories can be interpreted differently. The words Mutual Aid have been used to describe an anarchistic concept by Peter Kropotkin (1902), the coming together of people in self-help groups independent of skilled professionals' aid by Thomasina Borkman (1999), and more recently as a form of neighbourly activity during the COVID-19 pandemic.

Across the country, we've seen a huge outpouring of kindness during the covid-19 pandemic. In many communities, neighbours have organised themselves into mutual aid groups to support each other through lockdown. (Action Together, 2022)

To illustrate where volunteering takes place through organisations, we will use the categories in the Community Life Survey, a nationally representative annual survey of adults in England over 16 years of age, commissioned by the UK Department for Digital, Culture, Media and Sport. The Community Life Survey asks *"Have you been involved with any of the following groups, clubs or organisations during the last 12 months?"* (Department for Digital, Culture, Media and Sport, 2020a). We have added some examples, but we do not suggest any priority or preference beyond illustration. The examples are not comprehensive, and we have not captured the wide range of activities in community or neighbourhood groups. Volunteer involvement of any of these types can take many different forms, such as regular involvement expending much time or as short-term, one-off occasions, or even delivered online. It can happen locally, regionally, nationally and internationally.

1.2.1 Children's Education, Schools

Most parents will encounter volunteers when their children go to school and they might be invited to volunteer themselves. Wilkinson and Long (2019) in a Briefing Paper for the House of Commons Library estimate that there are currently around 300,000 school governors in England, 23,000 school governors in Wales and over 11,000 school governors in Northern Ireland while a membership body for Parent and Teacher Associations, 'Parentkind', reported that in 2020, it had 12,770 member organisations whose Committee members collectively volunteered 2.05 million hours (Parentkind, 2021).

1.2.2 Youth, Children's Activities, Outside School

Young people in school and outside of school are being encouraged to volunteer. The Youth Hostel Association in England and Wales website states that it offers many volunteering opportunities (Youth Hostel Association, 2022) suitable for volunteering as part of The Duke of Edinburgh Award scheme, involving 330,000 young people in 2020–2021 (Duke of Edinburgh's Award, 2021).

1.2.3 Adult Education

For people who want to continue to learn after school and widen their horizons and increase their knowledge through life-long education, volunteer involving organisations provide opportunities. The Workers' Educational Association (2022) is supported by nearly 2000 volunteers, while the Prince's Trust Group (2021) reports supporting 46,834 young people during 2020–2021 thanking the "*thousands of volunteers give their time freely to nurture and develop our young people*" (p. 57).

1.2.4 Sport, Exercise, Taking Part, Coaching or Going to Watch

Sport is arguably the largest area for volunteer involvement. A report to Sport England estimated that 15% of the adult population in England volunteered in sports (Taylor et al., 2003, p. 15) and in its Strategy for 'Volunteering in an Active Nation', Sport England (2016) states that 5.6 million people volunteer every month in sport and physical activity in England (p. 5).

1.2.5 Religion

For some, volunteering is part of their religious belief and undertaken as part of, or alongside worship. According to the 2019 annual review of the 'Jewish volunteering network', around 1000 people registered on its website in 2018 (Jewish Volunteering Network, 2019). 'Islamic Relief Worldwide' (2020) involves volunteers in a range of volunteering programmes, and the Church of England (2022) reports 23 million volunteering hours every month of "*community action over and above their normal church activities*".

1.2.6 Politics

Democracies cannot function without those volunteering to make them succeed. According to the Local Government Information Unit (2022), there are approximately 20,000 councillors in England, 1,277 in Scotland and 462 in Northern Ireland and of course local constituency parties rely on volunteers canvassing and supporting during elections and running local parties.

1.2.7 Older People

Older people affect volunteering and are affected by volunteering both as volunteers who assist people such as on helplines, but also as older volunteers engaging distinctively with volunteering and as beneficiaries. In their Annual Report Age, UK speak of their 7,500 volunteers supporting older people (Age UK, 2021, p. 52) and the Centre for Ageing Better (2020) suggests an "*inclusive approach to engaging older volunteers*".

1.2.8 Health, Disability and Social Welfare

Volunteering in health and social care has a longstanding tradition. Researchers of the King's Fund have estimated that three million people volunteer in health and social care across England (Naylor, 2013). This includes a wide range of organisations and opportunities such as hospital visiting, respite care, disability groups, medical research charities or providing emotional support such as though the Samaritans or NSPCC. There are also a variety of self-help groups such as Alcoholics Anonymous.

1.2.9 Safety, First Aid

Communal safety and first responding is often initiated by and relies on volunteer involvement. The Royal National Lifeboat Institution (2020) reports that *"Around 95% of RNLI people are volunteers—including around 5,600 crew members, 3,500 shore crew (including station management) and 140 lifeguards. About 23,000 other dedicated volunteers raise funds and awareness, give water safety advice and help in our museums, shops and offices"* (p. 5). The St John's Ambulance (2021) with an *"adult health volunteer community of around 11,000 people"* (p. 10) and British Red Cross (2021) which involves *"2,000 regular volunteers in the UK, over 88,000 community reserve volunteers"* (p. 10), offer a range of volunteering activities to people within their communities across the UK, including support at sports events such as football matches.

1.2.10 The Environment, Animal Welfare

A variety of volunteer involving organisations support and enable the conservation and environment sector, from small local to international, offering hands on practical opportunities. The Conservation Volunteers (2020), for example, set out the strategy to support 5,000 community groups. There are of course also groups of more disparate individuals such as Insulate Britain (2022) who come together for a common purpose, in their case to campaign for insulating all social housing in Britain by 2025.

1.2.11 Justice and Human Rights

In the criminal justice system, all 43 Home Office police forces together involve 9,174 volunteers as Special Constables (College of Policing, 2022a) and 8,014 as Police Support Volunteers (College of Policing, 2022b). The Magistrates Association (2020) reports that there are 13,177 magistrates, which are also called Justices of the Peace, who hear cases in court in their communities. There are also a variety of organisations supporting social justice initiatives such as community or race relations and LGBTQ+ groups. Amnesty International (2022) encourages people to volunteer for them and *"be part of a global movement standing together for human rights across the world"*. Citizens Advice (2022) report that they involve over *"20,000 volunteers including 17,000 who are invaluable to delivering our advice service and 2,200 in the Witness Service"*.

1.2.12 Local Community or Neighbourhood Groups

Volunteer involvement is intrinsic to community and neighbourhood activity. Nottingham Trent University research found falling membership levels in Neighbourhood Watch schemes which in 2017 was at 2.2 million households (Tseloni & Tura, 2019). However, during the COVID-19 pandemic of 2020–2022, many local community and neighbourhood groups emerged and became more visible (McCabe et al., 2021).

1.2.13 Citizens' Groups

Citizens' groups are by definition voluntary associations to promote citizenship. In its Report and Financial Statements, the National Federation of Women's Institutes of England, Wales, Jersey, Guernsey and the Isle of Man (2021) reported that it has 190,000 members in 5,500 Women's Institutes. It states as one of its four main purposes *"to advance citizenship for the public benefit by the promotion of civic responsibility and volunteering"* (p. 1). Rotary Clubs in Great Britain and Ireland report over 40,000 members who *"promote peace, fight disease, provide clean water, sanitation, and hygiene, save mothers and children, support education, grow local economies, protect the environment…"* (Rotary, 2022).

1.2.14 Hobbies, Recreation, Arts, Social Clubs

Volunteer involvement underpins a great many social recreational activities. A popular online volunteer matching tool advertised the following volunteering opportunity: *"Opportunities to act, dance, sing on stage…"*

(Do IT, 2022) and the Bluebell Railway (2021, 2022), a heritage steam railway line, offers more than 50 volunteering activities ranging from volunteering in "*Carriage and Wagon Works*" and "*Catering*" to "*Loco Works*" and the "*Museum*".

1.2.15 Trade Union Activity

Trade Union activities, not undertaken by paid staff, largely seem to fall within our definition of volunteering, as one union states: "*Members volunteer and train to support their colleagues, they contribute through discussion groups to shape the views and the opinions of the union, and they influence the responses made on their behalf*" (Community Trade Union, 2021). But there are questions around whether union members perceive themselves as volunteers and some trade unions clearly state that they do not accept volunteers as members (Unison, n.d.).

By using categories to characterise volunteering activities, we do not suggest that volunteering within a certain category necessarily reflects a shared or single vision of the volunteers or of the organisations involving volunteers. Indeed, volunteers and volunteer involving organisations within any one of the categories might well have differing purposes or even have opposing goals. Also, some volunteers or volunteer involving organisations that match those categories might not identify themselves as such.

Exploring volunteering undertaken by individuals and not through any volunteer involving organisation, the Community Life Survey also asks what unpaid help an individual may have given to other people: "*that is apart from any help given through a group, club or organisation. This could be help for a friend, neighbour or someone else but not a relative*" (Department for Digital, Culture, Media and Sport, 2020a). The survey suggests the following examples of where and how this may take place, but also recognises that there are many other forms not listed:

- babysitting or caring for children,
- giving advice,

- sitting with or providing personal care, such as washing, dressing, for someone who is sick or frail,
- cooking, cleaning, laundry, gardening or other routine household jobs,
- keeping in touch with someone who has difficulty getting out and about by visiting in person, telephoning or e-mailing,
- transporting or escorting someone to a hospital or on an outing,
- decorating, or any kind of home or car repairs,
- looking after a property or a pet for someone who is away,
- writing letters or filling in forms,
- shopping, collecting pension or paying bills,
- representing someone, talking to a council department or to a doctor.

Most volunteer involvement, including that which isn't undertaken through an organisation, does not just simply happen. Some forms of framework, structure and organising are often helpful to support it, even in self-organised community settings. We will explore this in the next section. But first, please consider your own views on how volunteering should be organised, by whom, when and what for? As before, we suggest turning the question on its head, in Exercise 1.3, considering whether there are occasions when volunteer involvement should not be organised or whether there are certain organisations which should not involve volunteers.

Exercise 1.3
- Who shouldn't be organising volunteering and why not?
- Maybe consider sections of the voluntary and community sector, the public sector, the private sector, uniformed services, essential services, secret services?

1.3   Involving Volunteers

Everyday, millions of people are volunteering. How do they find opportunities to volunteer, how do they know what needs doing and what can be done, and how do they know when to be at the right place and do things that make a difference? Volunteers and those who involve them carry out many complex activities and build different relationships. Volunteer involvement can be just between volunteers, or between volunteers and those who seek to involve them in delivering goals for an organisation. Reflecting on volunteer involvement therefore includes identifying when and how volunteers choose to become involved and what organisations who want to involve them might need to consider.

When we use the term 'involvement' in this book, we may also encapsulate concepts such as 'participation', 'engagement' and 'management'. These are often used interchangeably but all of them are contested and could even be interpreted with opposing meanings. Participation tends to mean 'taking part' whereas engagement is often used meaning 'receiving information or interacting'. Management tends to mean volunteer involvement that is akin to HR practices. It is necessary, as in the definitions of volunteering given already, to make clear what is meant, who puts it forward and why, because here also, the way people describe volunteer involvement reflects their personal and also political ideologies. We encourage everyone to be especially vigilant in the way they are using these terms.

When we use 'volunteer involvement', we first acknowledge that volunteers have power and resources to make their own choice to volunteer. We refer to this as having 'agency'. Volunteer involvement for us therefore means that volunteers are not just the unquestioning recipients of instruction by those who seek to involve them but have choice in the decisions about their volunteering and are partners in relationships. As this can take many forms, we must again be careful to describe the context and purpose of the various ways volunteers become involved.

1.3.1 On Not Using 'Formal' or 'Informal' Volunteering

We will not be using the terms 'formal volunteering' and 'informal volunteering' in this book and we recommend you don't. Even though these terms are commonly used, we think they can be misleading. However, we will leave the terms in the text if they are used in direct quotes. Next we explain why.

The Community Life Survey and many observers use the terms 'formal' and 'informal' to distinguish two main forms of volunteer involvement:

- volunteering through organisations such as clubs or charities and
- volunteering arranged by volunteers themselves.

However, volunteering arranged by volunteers themselves can still be formal. The groups they form may have written or unwritten rules and contact details for all members. Alternatively, volunteering through organisations could be informal without a need to register or to complete training. Likewise, much of the volunteering through organisations is arranged by volunteers themselves, in groups and associations without staff which are often not even registered. Additionally, some volunteer involvement infrastructure organisations are supporting processes to enable volunteering arranged by volunteers themselves in order to increase community-led volunteering to emerge, such as through fundraising baking sales, support groups or 'compassionate communities'. Even the Community Life Covid re-contact survey from 2020 found that people volunteering within the COVID-19 mutual aid groups counted this as formal despite mutual aid more commonly being considered informal (Department for Digital, Culture, Media and Sport, 2020b). This is further illustrated by the Scotland report on COVID-19, which found that there were a variety of structures of mutual aid groups, some loosely organised and spontaneously formed and others with much more structured operating models.

> This definition of 'mutual aid' highlights the limitations in the notion that volunteering can be clearly identified as being either 'formal' or 'informal'. (Scottish Government, 2022)

1.3.2 Organisations Involving Volunteers

Most volunteer involvement through volunteer involving organisations is arranged by volunteers themselves, as the majority of charities and not-for-profit organisations have no paid staff.

> It is estimated that only 9% of charities employ paid staff, while 91% are solely reliant on volunteers. (National Council for Voluntary Organisations, 2014, p. 4)

There are also many mostly small local voluntary groups not registered as charities or otherwise legally constituted, for which all activities are carried out on a voluntary basis. In comparison, the 9% of charities with paid staff are mostly larger volunteer involving organisations, and could have paid staff to coordinate and facilitate volunteering. This might be simply an addition to other duties carried out in someone's role or there may be a dedicated Volunteering Team. So for instance, the National Trust (2021, p. 20), reports that it involves 50,000 volunteers who may greet visitors, care for collections and clean parks. Attracting, connecting, training, supporting and thanking such a large number of volunteers, in many properties across the country, requires well-planned infrastructure and effort. Records need to be kept, rotas to be disseminated, problems to be dealt with. The role of staff supporting this form of volunteer involvement is to influence strategic decisions, to develop and maintain the logistics for involving volunteers, and also to coordinate the day-to-day experience and be the regular point of contact for volunteers. These elements could be incorporated within one staff role, or carried out by different posts as when a fundraising manager involves volunteer committees.

Yet, even in these larger organisations, volunteer involvement might be carried out through a branch network structure linked to a central organisation. One such is a federated structure, with local branches being independent local entities and others constituted as part of the whole organisation. As Davis Smith (1998) explains "*over a third (38%) of volunteers in the voluntary sector are involved with a branch of a supra-local organisation*" and a study of branches and networks of UK-wide charities carried out in 2000 identified that "*branches/groups in 73% of networks are run entirely by volunteers, 5% by paid staff, and 22% by a combination of both*" (Cited in Wyper, 2001, p. 32).

In some organisations, such as Samaritans and Scouts, day-to-day volunteer involvement is carried out by volunteers alongside or independently of paid staff. The paid staff team may lead on the development of tools and resources to enable volunteer leaders to volunteer in this capacity, and offer support with aspects of the experience journey, such as managing difficult conversations. Research carried out by NCVO in 2019 finds that volunteers with an unpaid coordinator are more likely to feel that the skills and experience which they wanted to use were used and less likely to feel that their volunteering was becoming too much like paid work than those who had a paid coordinator (McGarvey et al., 2019a). NCVO's research also demonstrated that key aspects for volunteers' satisfaction included feeling supported and recognised. At the same time, volunteers with no coordinator were least likely to feel well supported, which emphasises the need for some degree of structured involvement.

Of course, volunteering also takes place in organisations outside the voluntary and community sector, including those which are statutory, within local or central government, albeit not in equal numbers. Volunteering in the public sector at 17%, is a smaller proportion than within the not-for-profit sector which is 67% (McGarvey et al., 2020, p. 4). Volunteering in the public sector includes a wide range of opportunities, from sitting as a magistrate, volunteering with the police service, up to well over 50 activities in hospitals and community settings in health and social care (NHS England, 2017, p. 5), and increasingly supporting the provision of local authority responsibility such as in libraries. However, people volunteering within statutory services may not realise that this is the sector they are involved in (McGarvey et al., 2020, p.14). To add further to the confusion, many public services are actually carried out by charities. For example, the rehabilitation charity NACRO helps to run probation services and St John's Ambulance rather than an NHS ambulance could respond to a 999 emergency call (Slawson, 2016).

In yet another sector, many businesses and corporate companies recognise the benefit of volunteering as part of their corporate social responsibility and recognise a link between volunteering and their employees' morale and personal development. They are increasingly moving towards offering their staff time out of their usual working day to volunteer, as employer supported volunteering which can be described as follows:

> Employer-supported volunteering [ESV] provides employees the opportunity to volunteer with support from their employer, whether this is in the form of time off for individual volunteering or in a programme developed by the employer such as a team challenge event or ongoing arrangement with a community partner. (Volunteering England, 2011 cited in Grotz et al., 2021)

Employer-supported volunteering, sometimes known as corporate volunteering, makes up a smaller element of volunteer involvement with only 10% of volunteers saying that they are active this way (McGarvey et al., 2019a). However, following observations relating to people who were furloughed during the COVID-19 pandemic, there were calls to look at how this could be enabled more effectively, including recommendations to Government suggesting how this could be supported.

> As many of the people who have volunteered during furlough now return to work, these platforms—plugged into the Volunteer Passport database—could ensure the supply of assistance does not dry up, by helping people perform small-scale acts of voluntary service around their work commitments. (Kruger, 2020, p. 31)

While Kruger's associated suggestion of a National Volunteer Passport has been viewed as not likely to remove barriers and so has not been pursued by Department for Digital, Culture, Media and Sport (2022), employer-supported volunteering is found in all industries and sectors from the rail industry (Grotz et al., 2021) to community businesses, where numbers are particularly high.

> Latest figures suggest that there are nearly four times as many volunteers as paid staff involved in UK community businesses, with approximately 148,700 people giving their time to help out. (Higton et al., 2021)

Some organisations facilitate the involvement of volunteers rather than involve volunteers themselves. They are often referred to as 'volunteer infrastructure organisations' which act as brokers to help people to find volunteering opportunities, assist organisations to find volunteers, provide information on volunteer involvement and might run their own activities involving volunteers. Volunteer infrastructure organisations can also provide a role in connecting and enabling capacity building support including training on managing volunteers.

They include Councils for Voluntary Service, and Volunteer Centres and can be found not just in the voluntary but also the public and even private sectors. The London School of Economic and Political Science (LSE), for example, runs its own Volunteer Centre aiming to ensure that *"Every LSE student has the opportunity to volunteer"* and that *"LSE students are offered diverse volunteering opportunities from a broad range of organisations"* (London School of Economic and Political Science Volunteer Centre, 2022).

When comparing across volunteer involving organisations, most volunteer involvement, like with volunteering, is therefore carried out independently of constituted organisations, often by individuals on their own but also through bringing together people into communities, such as in Mutual Aid groups. Mutual Aid was happening in communities prior to the pandemic and hits the headlines periodically, as after Hurricane Sandy in 2012 in the United States, Mutual Aid group Occupy Sandy (Preston & Firth, 2020). Rochester (1999) points out that in such groups, volunteers might both assist others and receive assistance at the same time. Creating and facilitating a group of people in such ways is involving volunteers.

The size and complexity of the required efforts in volunteer involvement depends mostly on the number of volunteers, and also on the nature of their volunteering. There is a great deal of difference between specialist volunteers who have been extensively trained, like RNLI lifeboat crew members and people taking on ad hoc tasks not requiring specific skills, like volunteers taking part in an annual litter pick.

1.4   How Many People Volunteer and Why?

Despite the uncertainty regarding terms and the confusion this causes, we can find estimates of how many people volunteer. The latest report of the United Nations on volunteering, the 2022 State of the Worlds Volunteering Report suggests that the total number of volunteers globally in 2021 may exceed 3 billion (United Nations Volunteers Programme, 2021). In the UK, it is thought that around 70% of people have volunteered sometime in their lives (McGarvey et al., 2019b) and according to the Citizenship Survey, 2001–2011 and the Community Life Survey, 2012–2022 overall numbers of volunteers have broadly stayed the same for the last 20 years. However, numbers have been falling slightly since the year of the London Olympics and Paralympics and of course they were impacted by the COVID-19 pandemic, see Fig. 1.1.

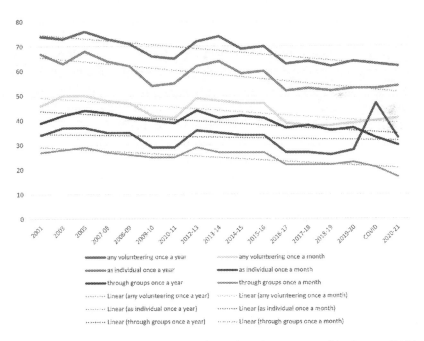

Fig. 1.1 'Volunteer numbers' is based on data from Citizenship Survey (2001–2011) and Community Life Survey (2012–2021)

Based on findings from these repeated surveys, we can be confident that nearly three quarters of all people in England volunteer at times. More of them volunteer as individuals and not through organisations but about one in four regularly volunteer through volunteer involving organisations. During the COVID-19 pandemic, we saw a spike in volunteering as an 'individual once a month' but that now also appears to be returning to pre-pandemic levels. While trends of all forms of volunteering appear to be falling slightly since this survey began in 2001, about one-third of the people appear to have continued to regularly volunteer as individuals throughout.

Yet, these numbers hide many differences. In England, education and socio-economic status would seem to be the most notable characteristics influencing whether people are likely to say that they volunteer, suggesting that educated people from higher socio-economic groups are more likely to volunteer than others. This also indicates that some people and groups might find it easier than others to volunteer in certain ways. NCVO's Time Well Spent survey describes many of these differences and recognises that people from all diverse backgrounds volunteer, but confirms a less positive experience for some demographics, due to a lack of flexibility and attitudes of other volunteers (Donahue et al., 2020, p. 4). This can also be seen in the context that volunteering is not just a modern Western concept and has roots in many societies around the globe including many religions (Lukka et al., 2003), which do not appear to feature in the main discourses. Likewise, while exclusion from volunteering has been well recognised for decades (Institute for Volunteering Research, 2004), this does not seem to have been significantly challenged. In light of such challenging findings and in particular more recently wider social movements such as Black Lives Matter, considerations around equity, diversity and inclusion have gained prominence within organisations involving volunteers. We will discuss this in Chapter 3, on critical perspectives.

We close this chapter by considering why people volunteer. Before we do, we suggest you consider people's motivations to volunteer and what you find to be acceptable motivations and reasons why. To help to do this, you can again turn this question on its head by asking yourself what you find unacceptable. See Exercise 1.4.

Exercise 1.4

Is it ok to volunteer for fun or my own benefit? Is it ok to volunteer to:

- get a job?
- get a jab?
- get a date?
- to stop people from getting jobs?
- to stop people from getting jabs?
- to organise fights?

Reflecting on the examples above what motivations do you think people have when they volunteer and what motivations would you find **unacceptable.**
Why would those motivations be unacceptable to you?

In 2007, the Cabinet Office funded a national survey to ask people about their motivations to start volunteering. "*I wanted to improve things, help people*" came out as the top reason (Low et al., 2007, p. 34). That survey question offered a range of other motivations which were rated in the following order 'help people', 'cause was important to me', 'I had time to spare', 'I wanted to meet people, make friends', 'connected with needs, interests of family or friends', 'there was a need in the community', 'to use existing skills', 'part of my philosophy of life' 'friends, family did it', 'to learn new skills', 'part of my religious belief', 'no one else to do it' 'to help get on in my career', 'had received voluntary help myself', 'to get a recognised qualification', 'already involved in the organisation', 'connected with my interests, hobbies' and 'to give something back' (Low et al., 2007, pp. 34–37). Volunteers have different motivations, partly depending on characteristics such as age. The motivation 'to help get on in my career' is found more frequently among 16–24 year olds, whereas 'I had spare time' was unsurprisingly highest among those over 65 years old and possibly retired (Low et al., 2007, p. 36). The question why volunteers continue to volunteer can also be linked to volunteer's motivation, and here the strongest reason appears to be having had good volunteering experience.

> How volunteers feel about their volunteering experience is most strongly associated with overall satisfaction—over and above 'who they are'. (McGarvey et al., 2019b, p. 55)

Unfortunately, although it is not often mentioned, and not generally explored in surveys, people may also have suspect or nefarious motivations. People with negative intentions might become volunteers to get access to vulnerable people and this is why organisations connecting volunteers with vulnerable people will undertake background checks. However, there are many more reasons for people to volunteer, on a spectrum from outright altruistic, to self-serving and in the extreme, criminal. We must take this into account when we discuss volunteer involvement and we shall explore this further in Chapter 3.

1.5   Summary and Conclusions

In this chapter, we have explored the complexity of volunteer involvement, encouraging you to reflect on the way you use the words 'volunteering' and 'involvement' and to consider your own views about them. We described how for us, 'volunteer involvement' is about the relationships established so as to attain shared goals in which all those involved have agency and choice. This reflects how we separately see 'volunteering' and 'involvement', and how we understand and view the contexts in which these relationships take place.

References

Action Together. (2022). *What is a mutual aid group?* Explanation on Action Together webpages for Oldham, Rochdale and Tameside. https://www.act iontogether.org.uk/mutual-aid#1. Accessed 27 August 2022.

Age UK. (2021). *Helping the older people who need us the most, a pandemic year—Rising to the challenge: Age UK Report of Trustees and Annual Accounts 2020/21.* Age UK. https://www.ageuk.org.uk/globalassets/age-uk/docume nts/annual-reports-and-reviews/age-uk-annual-report-2021.pdf. Accessed 26 June 2022.

Amnesty International. (2022). *Together we are powerful.* Page on the website of Amnesty International. https://www.amnesty.org/en/get-involved/. Accessed 27 June 2022.

Beveridge, L. (1948). *Voluntary action.* George Allen & Unwin Ltd.

Bluebell Railway. (2021). *Trust & society combined report & accounts 2021.* Bluebell Railway. https://www.bluebell-railway.co.uk/bluebell/soc/notices/trust_ brps_accounts_only.pdf. Accessed 27 June 2022.

Bluebell Railway. (2022). *Volunteer at Bluebell Railway.* Page on the Bluebell Railway website. https://www.bluebell-railway.com/volunteer-at-bluebell-rai lway/. Accessed 27 June 2022.

Borkman, T. (1999). *Understanding self-help/mutual aid: Experiential learning in the commons.* Rutgers University Press.

British Red Cross. (2021). *Trustees' report and accounts.* British Red Cross. https://www.redcross.org.uk/about-us/how-we-are-run/our-finances/ annual-reports-and-accounts. Accessed 26 June 2022.

Citizens Advice. (2022). *Volunteering with citizens advice.* Page on the website of Citizens Advice. https://www.citizensadvice.org.uk/about-us/support-us/ volunteering/. Accessed 27 June 2022.

Centre for Ageing Better. (2020). *Helping out: Taking an inclusive approach to engaging older volunteers.* Centre for Aging Better. https://ageing-better.org. uk/sites/default/files/2021-08/Helping-out-engaging-older-volunteers.pdf. Accessed 26 June 2022.

Church of England. (2022). *Managing volunteers.* Webpage on the Church of England website. https://www.churchofengland.org/resources/commun ity-action/managing-volunteers. Accessed 26 June 2022.

Cnaan, R., Handy, F., & Wadsworth, M. (1996). Defining who is a volunteer: Conceptional and empirical considerations. *Nonprofit and Voluntary Sector Quarterly, 23,* 335–351.

College of Policing. (2022a). *Special constables*. College of Policing. https://www.college.police.uk/guidance/special-constables. Accessed 27 June 2022.

College of Policing. (2022b). *Police support volunteers*. College of Policing. https://www.college.police.uk/guidance/involving-citizens-policing/police-support-volunteers. Accessed 27 June 2022.

Commission on the Future of Volunteering. (2008). *Report of the commission on the future of volunteering and manifesto for change*. Volunteering England.

Community Trade Union. (2021). *What is a trade union*. Page on the website of Community Trade Union last updated 15 November 2021. https://community-tu.org/who-we-are/what-is-a-trade-union/. Accessed 27 June 2022.

Conservation Volunteers. (2020). *For people and green spaces: A thriving network for everyone: Strategy 2021–25*. The Conservation Volunteers. https://www.tcv.org.uk/wp-content/uploads/2021/07/Strategy_brochure_visual-final-singles.pdf. Accessed 27 June 2022.

Davis Smith, J. (1998). *The 1997 national survey of volunteering*. Institute for Volunteering Research.

Department for Culture Media and Sport. (n.d.). *Enabling social action section A: A description of social action*. Department for Culture Media and Sport and New Economics Foundation. https://assets.publishing.service.gov.uk/government/uploads/system/uploads/attachment_data/file/591797/A_description_of_social_action.pdf. Accessed 26 June 2022.

Department for Digital, Culture, Media and Sport. (2020a). *Community life survey technical report 2019/20*. Department for Digital, Culture, Media and Sport.

Department for Digital, Culture, Media and Sport. (2020b). *3. Formal volunteering—Community life COVID-19 re-contact survey 2020*. Department for Digital, Culture, Media and Sport. https://www.gov.uk/government/statistics/community-life-covid-19-re-contact-survey-2020-main-report/3-formal-volunteering-community-life-recontact-survey-2020. Accessed 27 August 2022.

Department for Digital, Culture, Media and Sport. (2022). *Government response to Danny Kruger MP's report: 'Levelling up our communities: Proposals for a new social covenant*. Page on the website of the Department for Digital, Culture, Media & Sport. https://www.gov.uk/government/publications/government-response-to-danny-kruger-mps-report-levelling-up-our-communities-proposals-for-a-new-social-covenant/government-response-to-danny-kruger-mps-report-levelling-up-our-communities-proposals-for-a-new-social-covenant. Accessed 27 August 2022.

Do IT. (2022). *Amateur dramatics.* Page on the website of Do IT. https://doit. life/volunteering-opportunity/md/28778. Accessed 27 June 2022.

Donahue, K., McGarvey, A., Rooney, K., & Jochum, V. (2020). *Time well Spent: Diversity and volunteering research report December 2020.* National Council for Voluntary Organisations. https://ncvo-app-wagtail-mediaa721 a567-uwkfinin077j.s3.amazonaws.com/documents/time_well_spent_divers ity_and_volunteering_final.pdf. Accessed 28 August 2022]

Duke of Edinburgh's Award. (2021). *Annual report and financial statements for the year ended 31 March 2021.* Duke of Edinburgh's Award. https://www.dofe.org/wp-content/uploads/2022/01/JC0375_DofE-Annual-Report_27_01_21.pdf. Accessed 26 June 2022.

Grotz, J. (2011). *Divisive, harmful and fatal: Less recognised impacts of volunteering.* Paper delivered at the NCVO/VSSN "Researching the Voluntary Sector" Conference 7–8 September 2011, London.

Grotz J., Birt, L., Edwards, H., Locke M., & Poland F. (2021, February). Exploring disconnected discourses about patient and public involvement and volunteer involvement in English health and social care. *Health Expect, 24*(1), 8–18. https://doi.org/10.1111/hex.13162. Epub 2020 Dec 1. PMID: 33259704; PMCID: PMC7879540.

Higton, J., Archer, R., Merrett, D., Hansel, M., & Howe, P. (2021). *The community business market in 2020* (Research Institute Report No. 29). London: Power to Change.

Home Office. (2021). *Permission to work and volunteering for asylum seekers Version 10.0.* Home Office. https://assets.publishing.service.gov.uk/govern ment/uploads/system/uploads/attachment_data/file/983283/permission-to-work-v10.0ext.pdf. Accessed 28 August 2022.

Hustinx, L., Cnaan, R. A., & Handy, F. (2010). Navigating theories of volunteering: A hybrid map for a complex phenomenon. *Journal for the Theory of Social Behaviour, 40*(4), 410–434. https://doi.org/10.1111/j.1468-5914. 2010.00439.x

Institute for Volunteering Research. (2004). *Volunteering for all: Exploring the link between volunteering and social exclusion.* Institute for Volunteering Research. https://www.bl.uk/collection-items/volunteering-for-all-exploring-the-link-between-volunteering-and-social-exclusion. Accessed 1 September 2022.

Insulate Britain. (2022). *Help support the Insulate Britain Campaign.* Homepage of insulatebritain.com. http://insulatebritain.com. Accessed 27 June 2022.

Islamic Relief Worldwide. (2020). *Annual report and financial statements.* Islamic Relief Worldwide. https://www.islamic-relief.org.uk/wp-content/upl oads/2021/08/IRW-AnnualReport2020-Signed.pdf. Accessed 26 June 2022.

Jewish Volunteering Network. (2019). *Annual review 2018–2019.* Jewish Volunteering Network. https://www.jvn.org.uk/files/?m=3255&s=1&l=1. Accessed 26 June 2022.

Kearney J. (2001). The values and basic principles of volunteering: Complacency or caution? *Voluntary Action, 3*(3), 63–86. Reprinted in Davis-Smith, J., & Locke, M. (Eds.). (2007). *Volunteering and the test of time: Essays for policy, organisation and research.* Institute for Volunteering Research.

Kropotkin, P. (1902). *Mutual aid: A factor of evolution.* Heineman.

Kruger, D. (2020). *Levelling up our communities: Proposals for a new social covenant A report for government by Danny Kruger MP.* A report posted on the website of Danny Kruger MP. https://www.dannykruger.org.uk/files/ 2020-09/Kruger%202.0%20Levelling%20Up%20Our%20Communities. pdf. Accessed 26 June 2022.

Local Government Information Unit. (2022). *Local government facts and figures: England.* Webpage on the website of the Local Government Information Unit. https://lgiu.org/local-government-facts-and-figures-england/#sec tion-4. Accessed 26 June 2022.

London School of Economic and Political Science Volunteer Centre. (2022). *About the LSE volunteer centre: Vision, mission and outcomes 2017–22.* Page on the Website of the London School of Economic and Political Science. https://info.lse.ac.uk/current-students/volunteer-centre/About-us. Accessed 26 June 2022.

Low, N., Butt, S., Ellis Paine, A., & Davis-Smith, J. (2007). *Helping out: A national survey of volunteering and charitable giving.* Cabinet Office.

Lukka, P., & Locke, M., with Soteri-Procter, A. (2003). *Faith and voluntary action: Community, values and resources.* Institute for Volunteering Research.

Magistrates Association. (2020). *Statistics published on diversity in the magistracy.* Page on the website of the Magistrates Association posted 29 September 2020. https://www.magistrates-association.org.uk/News-and-comments/statistics-published-on-diversity-in-the-magistracy. Accessed 27 June 2022.

McCabe, A., Wilson, M., Macmillan, R., & Ellis Paine, A. (2021). *Now they see us: Communities responding to COVID-19.* Report on the website of the Local Trust. https://localtrust.org.uk/wp-content/uploads/2021/07/ Now-they-see-us.pdf. Accessed 25 June 2022.

McGarvey, A., Jochum, V., & Chan, O. (2019a). *Time well spent: Employer-supported volunteering* (Research Report). London: National Council for Voluntary Organisations. https://www.befriending.co.uk/resources/24751-time-well-spent-employer-supported-volunteering. Accessed 27 August 2022.

McGarvey, A., Jochum, V., Chan, O., Delaney, S., Young, R., & Gillies, C. (2020). *Time well spent: Volunteering in the public sector* (Research Report). London: National Council for Voluntary Organisations. https://www.befriending.co.uk/r/24836-time-well-spent-volunteering-in-the-public-sector. Accessed 27 August 2022.

McGarvey, A., Jochum, V., Davies, J., Dobbs, J., & Hornung, L. (2019b). *Time well spent: A national survey on the volunteer experience.* NCVO.

Naylor, C., Mundle, C., Weaks, L., & Buck, D. (2013). *Volunteering in health and care: Securing a sustainable Future.* Kings Fund. https://www.kingsfund.org.uk/sites/default/files/field/field_publication_file/volunteering-in-health-and-social-care-kingsfund-mar13.pdf. Accessed 26 June 2022.

National Council for Voluntary Organisations. (2014). *Report of the inquiry into charity senior executive pay.* National Council for Voluntary Organisations. https://www.ncvo.org.uk/images/news/Executive-Pay-Report.pdf. Accessed 27 June 2022.

National Trust. (2021). *Annual report 2020/21.* National Trust. https://nt.global.ssl.fastly.net/documents/annual-report-202021.pdf. Accessed 27 June 2022.

NHS England. (2017). *Recruiting and managing volunteers in NHS providers: A practical guide.* NHS England. https://www.england.nhs.uk/wp-content/uploads/2017/10/recruiting-managing-volunteers-nhs-providers-practical-guide.pdf. Accessed 4 August 2022.

Parentkind. (2021). *Report and accounts for the year ended 31 December 2020.* Parentkind.

Preston, J., & Firth, R. (2020). *Coronavirus, class and mutual aid in the United Kingdom.* Palgrave Macmillan.

Prince's Trust Group. (2021). *Annual report and accounts 2020/21.* Prince's Trust Group. https://www.princes-trust.org.uk/about-the-trust/research-policies-reports/annual-report. Accessed 28 June 2022.

Rochester, C. (1999). One size does not fit all: Four models of involving volunteers in small voluntary organisations. *Voluntary Action, 1*(2), 7–20.

Rotary. (2022). *About Rotary.* Page on Rotary Website. https://www.rotary.org/en/get-involved/rotary-clubs. Accessed 27 June 2022.

Royal National Lifeboat Institution. (2020). *RNLI annual report and accounts 2020: A year like no other*. Royal National Lifeboat Institution. https://rnli.org/about-us/how-the-rnli-is-run/annual-report-and-accounts. Accessed 26 June 2022.

Scottish Government. (2022). *Scotland's volunteering action plan*. Scottish Government. https://www.gov.scot/publications/scotlands-volunteering-action-plan/. Accessed 26 July 2022.

Slawson, N. (2016). *The public services you didn't know were run by charities*. News on The Guardian webpages published 20 May 2016. https://www.theguardian.com/voluntary-sector-network/2016/may/20/10-public-services-run-charities. Accessed 27 June 2022.

Smith, D. H., Stebbins, R. A., & Grotz, J. (Eds.). (2016). *The Palgrave handbook of volunteering, civic participation, and nonprofit associations*. Palgrave Macmillan.

Sport England. (2016). *Volunteering in an active nation*. Sport England. https://sportengland-production-files.s3.eu-west-2.amazonaws.com/s3fs-public/2020-01/volunteering-in-an-active-nation-final.pdf?VersionId=LU3cqHb9FZvVWi3rye.b.HNIe5UM9wOX. Accessed 26 June 2022.

St John Ambulance. (2021). *Humanity in crisis: Annual report and accounts for the year ended 31 December 2020*. St John Ambulance. https://www.sja.org.uk/globalassets/documents/annual-reports-and-accounts/st-john-ambulance-annual-report-2020_web.pdf. Accessed 26 June 2022.

Taylor, P., Nichols, G., Holmes, K., James, M., Gratton, C., Garrett, R., Kokolakakis, T., Mulder, C., & King, L. (2003). *Sports volunteering in England 2002: A report for Sports England*. Leisure Industries Research Centre. https://sportengland-production-files.s3.eu-west-2.amazonaws.com/s3fs-public/valuing-volunteering-in-sport-in-england-final-report.pdf. Accessed 26 June 2022.

Tseloni, A., & Tura, F. (2019). *Neighbourhood watch membership: Trends, obstacles, members' and potential members' profiles executive summary*. Nottingham Trent University. https://www.ourwatch.org.uk/sites/default/files/documents/2020-01/Neighbourhood%20Watch%20Membership%20exetutive%20summary.pdf. Accessed 27 June 2022.

Unison. (n.d.). *Volunteers*. Guidance on the website of Unison. https://www.unison.org.uk/content/uploads/2016/01/Volunteers.pdf. Accessed 5 August 2022.

United Nations General Assembly. (2001a). *UNGA Resolution 56/38: Recommendations on support for volunteering*. Page on website of UN Volunteers. https://www.unv.org/publications/unga-resolution-5638-recommendations-support-volunteering. Accessed 28 June 2022.

United Nations Volunteers (UNV) Programme. (2021). *2022 state of the world's volunteerism report. Building equal and inclusive societies*. United Nations Volunteers (UNV) programme.

Volunteering England. (2011). *The practical guide to employer supported volunteering for employers*. Volunteering England.

Wilkinson, N., & Long, R. (2019). *School governance: Briefing paper number 08072, 17 December 2019*. House of Commons Library. https://researchbriefings.files.parliament.uk/documents/CBP-8072/CBP-8072.pdf. Accessed 26 June 2022.

Wilson, J. (2000). Volunteering. *Annual Review of Sociology, 26*, 215–240.

Women's Institutes of England, Wales, Jersey, Guernsey and the Isle of Man. (2021). *Report and financial statements for the year ended 30 September 2021*. Women's Institutes of England, Wales, Jersey, Guernsey and the Isle of Man. https://www.thewi.org.uk/__data/assets/pdf_file/0008/569681/NFWI-Signed-Trustees-Annual-Return-for-September-2021.pdf. Accessed 27 June 2022.

Workers' Educational Association. (2022). *About us*. Webpages of the https://www.wea.org.uk/. https://www.wea.org.uk/about-us. Accessed 26 June 2022.

Wyper, H. (2001). *The outlook for branch/group networks of national charities: What can be learnt from a survey of relevant organisations?* [Dissertation]. Centre for Voluntary Sector and Not-for-Profit Management City University Business School.

Youth Hostel Association. (2022). *Complete your award with us DofE: Can we count you in?* Pages on https://volunteer.yha.org.uk/. https://volunteer.yha.org.uk/index-classic. Accessed 26 June 2022.

2

Historical and Conceptual Background

Abstract This chapter sets volunteer involvement in historical context, outlines how it is conceived, offers models of volunteer involvement and considers the plurality of volunteer involvement concepts, including the role of ideology and the state. It encourages the reader to use five 'Exercises' to reflect on how volunteering has changed over time, how it is conceptualised and organised today and who should have power to make decisions.

Keywords History · Plurality · Models

Volunteer involvement can be thought of in many different ways. Some characterise volunteers as 'do-gooders' or 'Lady Bountiful' while others see them as activists essential to changing the world. Some volunteers don't even describe themselves as volunteers and others see them as privileged people with colonial attitudes. These views of volunteering are also constantly changing or evolving. The initially sceptical journalist O'Hagan (2001) put together 15 case studies from Northern Ireland and then concluded "*I now think that the notion of do-gooders is a false*

© The Author(s), under exclusive license to Springer Nature
Switzerland AG 2022
J. Grotz and R. Leonard, *Volunteer Involvement*,
https://doi.org/10.1007/978-3-031-19221-0_2

idea born out of prejudice". The United Nations' approach to volunteering also changed, from transactional to participatory as it moved from suggesting at the beginning of the millennium that voluntary activities must support development goals (United Nations General Assembly, 2001) to explaining in 2021 how volunteering can help build equal and inclusive societies (United Nations Volunteers Programme, 2021).

In the UK, over the last two centuries, major achievements of volunteer involvement have been recorded and debated, as when the suffragette movement involved volunteers for events and *"collected names of local women prepared for arrest and sent these to Headquarters in advance so leaders could anticipate the scale of any planned action"* (Cowman, 2018). Around the globe, campaigns such as direct-action advocacy groups raise awareness for example of the HIV/AIDs epidemic and pressured governments into taking action. One of the effective methods of protest used by ACT UP groups was the mass 'die-in' which involved protestors lying on the ground completely still as though dead, often in the road and outside key buildings. (ACT UP London, 2022).

However, mistakes were also made, sometimes when the state became involved. A common mistake by governments, has been asking for large numbers of volunteers to help, but then not knowing how to involve them effectively, or lacking a good reason to do so. In 1917, the newly established British political and cultural magazine the New Statesman described why the scheme for National Service Volunteers was not getting off to a good start. Their description still resonates today, in view of more recent initiatives that encountered similar problems.

> In late 1916, Neville Chamberlain, …set up a scheme for National Service Volunteers to serve in the roles vacated by the men fighting in France and quickly amassed some 200,000 volunteers. What to do with them though?… Chamberlain had ignored the rules of supply and demand with the result that too few volunteers were set to useful work and the scheme was a "fiasco". Later in 1917, Chamberlain resigned. (New Statesman Archive, 2021)

We will now provide a brief historical overview of volunteering and volunteer involvement, consider different views of volunteer involvement and discuss the role of the state. To bring in your views and experience, please first consider the question in Exercise 2.1.

> **Exercise 2.1**
>
> When and how did volunteering begin?

2.1 A Very Short History of Volunteering and Volunteer Involvement

It may surprise you to learn that the former chief economist of the Bank of England, and at the time of writing this book, the UK Government's Chair of Levelling Up Advisory Council, Andy Haldane, reminds us that "*Our societies thrived for many, many millennia before anything recognisably like either the market or the state appeared on the scene*" (Haldane, 2021). Volunteering can be seen as a factor that enabled societies to thrive, long before the state and the market. While specific volunteering activities may not leave much trace, the groups that volunteers form might well do.

> Volunteering seems to be a characteristic of our species, with informal (unorganized) volunteering probably going back to our origins 150,000–200,000 years ago. Formal volunteering in associations can only be traced back about 10,000 years to the origins of associations in which to do such volunteering. (Harris et al., 2016, p. 23)

Throughout our recorded history, we can find a wide variety of forms of volunteering emerging which continue until today, for example:

- People sharing a belief getting together is prominent through volunteering in faith groups.
- People producing food together in agrarian societies is still seen in modern collective endeavours such as the co-operative movement.

- People finding themselves in similar disadvantaged situations. Long before modern movements, disabled people got together to form associations (Grotz, 1992).
- People getting together for mutual support within their trade, through guilds, still seen in today's trade unions.

And we can find examples everywhere around the globe with the earliest examples from the Americas, Australia, China, India, Mesopotamia, Greece and Rome, among others (Harris et al., 2016). From the Middle Ages, we have clearer evidence such as from the European merchant guilds and by the nineteenth century, volunteering in more structured bodies had become widespread in the UK, as Bourdillon (1945) describes so vividly in terms of shared enthusiasm, when discussing the place of voluntary social services in society:

> The habit of forming voluntary associations for every sort of social purpose is widely spread and deeply rooted in this country. Quite naturally in Britain when a man has a new enthusiasm he buys a twopenny notebook, prints 'Minute Book' carefully on the first page, calls together some of his friends under the name of a Committee – and behold a new voluntary society is launched. (p. 1)

At the beginning of the twentieth century, faith and mutual support, in religious congregations and friendly societies remained major drivers of such associations, and one specific purpose, to meet some of society's social needs, gained prominence. In the UK in 1919, several associations began to be organised nationally, in the National Council for Social Service, which became the present National Council for Voluntary Organisations (Davis Smith, 2019). At the same time, evidence grew of other forms of volunteering, such as volunteering for leisure and sport and volunteering for social change or conservation and protection, as well. Thus, the German Gymnasium, a listed building in London, and now a restaurant, was funded and used for sport by an association of the German Gymnastic Movement. It was even used for events during the 1866 London Olympian Games, the forerunner of the modern Olympics games (Barker, 2016; Volans, 2010).

In 1889, the Society for the Protection of Birds (RSPB) was created by a group of women frustrated because the British Ornithological Union did not pick up on the need to campaign against the use of feathers in fashion, challenging the status quo. In RSPB founder Emily Williamsons' words:

> Women are mostly timid in inaugurating anything, but they are very ready to give their help to a good cause when they are shown the way. (Royal Society for the Protection of Birds, 2022)

In the UK, the end of the Second World War brought fundamental changes to health and social care, and during the immediate post-war years, the involvement of volunteers changed. Health care, which had previously seen much volunteer involvement, saw an initial decrease when the governance of hospitals was nationalised as part of the formation of the NHS (Abel-Smith, 1964). However, instead of an expected reduced role for volunteering and volunteer involving organisations, the following decades saw their activities increase (Davis Smith et al., 1995) along with culture shifts. Such culture shifts are also seen as the foundation for developing the construct of volunteering as an alternative 'workforce'. Rochester (2013) describes how this can be followed through four consecutive committees or commissions. In the 60's, the Aves Committee considered the '*Voluntary Worker in the Social Services*' (Aves, 1969), followed in the 70's by the Wolfenden Committee (1978), the Commission on the Future of the Voluntary Sector (1996) led by Nicholas Deakin and the Commission on the Future of Volunteering (2008) led by Julia Neuberger. Internationally, following proposals from Japan, around the turn of the millennium, volunteering gained recognition from the United Nations as a major societal force, with the first international year of the volunteer being observed in 2001.

Before moving to the next section, which will consider different ways of conceptualising volunteering, please ask yourself the question in Exercise 2.2 about whether some forms of volunteering are better than others.

Exercise 2.2

Are some forms of volunteering better than others? Which volunteers deserve awards?

2.2   Conceiving Volunteering

The way we conceptualise volunteering influences what we volunteer for and how we volunteer. As a corollary, the way we volunteer also influences how we conceptualise it. There are at least five common but very different ways to think about volunteering as being for:

- someone else: philanthropic, service
- each other: mutual aid, co-operative
- oneself: leisure, advancement, social contacts
- democracy: participation
- change the world: campaigning

Again, these types are almost never clear-cut and often overlap. To emphasise how people have thought and continue to think about these types, we can first draw on two ideas from Beveridge's seminal post-war book on Voluntary Action, in which he used the concepts of the 'Mutual Aid Motive' and the 'Philanthropic Motive' (Beveridge, 1948). We will then discuss three types that have since been added to the debate: volunteering as 'leisure', 'participation' and 'campaigning'. We will also briefly address volunteering abroad which can span all five types but has its own issues. Finally, we consider what it means if people don't recognise their involvement as volunteering.

2.2.1 Volunteering for Someone Else

Beveridge (1948) describes the 'philanthropic motive' in the language of his time, linked to social conscience:

...the feeling which makes men who are materially comfortable, mentally uncomfortable so long as their neighbours are materially uncomfortable: to have social conscience is to be unwilling to make a separate peace with the giant social evils of Want, Disease, Squalor, Ignorance, Idleness, escaping into personal prosperity oneself, while leaving one's fellows in their clutches. (p. 9)

The United Nations Volunteers Programme (2021) presents this motivation as leading to volunteering as service: "*where volunteers respond to the perceived needs of another person or community*" (p. 19). Volunteering in this way is not necessarily undertaken to change the world and can be seen as part of maintaining the status quo. Today, choosing to be involved in this way is often described by volunteers themselves as 'wanting to give something back'. This form of volunteering is commonly observed when organisations that have a mission to address issues such as Beveridge's "*Want, Disease, Squalor, Ignorance, Idleness*" (1948, p. 9), involve volunteers to address these. In more current language, they could seek to address poverty, health, housing, education and unemployment. Volunteering involvement, here, tends to provide relief from the worst effects rather than challenge the causes of the issues. Again, an organisation's attitudes or strategic direction might change over time, as might the nature of their volunteer involvement. Even if this form of volunteering is seen more as being for others, there is strong evidence that it also benefits the volunteers.

2.2.2 Volunteering for Each Other

As an alternative, Beveridge (1948) derives the motive for mutual aid from thrift and self-interest:

a sense of one's own need for security against misfortune, and realisation that since one's fellow have the same need, by undertaking to help one another all may help themselves. (p. 9)

However, when referring to Mutual Aid, other authors and observers have interpreted those words very differently, not just compared with

Beveridge who looked at citizen organisations such as 'Friendly Societies', but also distinctly different from each other. Most recently Mutual Aid resonated with some of the activities reported during the COVID-19 crisis. On the website 'covidmutualaid.org', 'mutual aid' is described as:

> where a group of people organise to meet their own needs, outside of the formal frameworks of charities, NGOs and government. (COVID-19 Mutual Aid UK, 2022a)

Their activities are described as

> local community groups organising mutual aid throughout the Covid-19 outbreak .... providing resources and connecting people to their nearest local groups, to willing volunteers and to those in need. (COVID-19 Mutual Aid UK, 2022b)

Those using the words Mutual Aid in the context of the COVID-19 pandemic do not seem to draw on definitions from either Kropotkin (1902), or Borkman (1999) whose seminal books have 'Mutual Aid' in their title, but also interpret it differently.

Volunteering for each other, which characterises mutual aid, is commonly found in organisations with volunteers who share a similar problem or issue. They tend to focus on resolving this problem together, for and with their members. The United Nations Volunteers Programme (2021) describes it as:

> ...the wealth of informal, person-to-person helping activities embedded in community and cultural practices. People gather to volunteer together as a response to a shared need or issue. (p. 19)

2.2.3 Volunteering for Oneself

Unlike the first two, this form of volunteering is less ostensibly undertaken as helping others or each other and more for having fun doing what you like doing, most notably sport and hobbies. Stebbins and

Graham (2004) speak of 'volunteering as leisure and leisure as volunteering'. Sport England (2016) reports in its strategy that 5.6 million people volunteer every month in sport and physical activity in England (p. 5). In a reverse of the point made above, explaining that volunteering for others also benefits volunteers, the fact that this form of volunteering is predominantly undertaken for oneself, as leisure, does not mean that it doesn't also benefit others. Sport England (2016) cites the Office for National Statistics which estimates that the volunteering time is "*worth £24 billion, the equivalent of 1.5% of GDP*" (p. 5). Understanding the benefit to others can also be applied to steam engine enthusiasts whose hobby has ensured that we still have heritage railway tracks throughout the UK.

Volunteering for oneself can also be for personal advancement. When discussing education and employment, volunteering is regularly identified as a positive activity. In 2007, an Institute for Volunteering Research report for the Commission on the Future of Volunteering, cites a Timebank survey of companies which found "*that 94 per cent of respondents thought that volunteering added to the skills of their workforce*" (Ockenden, 2007). A later evaluation of students programme called 'Inspired', confirmed that "*enhancing employability is a major motivational factor for volunteering*" (Brewis et al., 2010, p. 114). It is nonetheless noteworthy, that research by the National Council for Voluntary Organisations (2018) found that while volunteering can improve both hard and soft skills, evidence is weak for volunteering actually leading to people finding paid employment.

2.2.4 Volunteering for Democracy

There are at least two ways to see this form of volunteering. Firstly, there is volunteering in civic roles, as lay members of the courts or youth offender panels, health watch, school governors and many more. Participation here has been described as "the backbone of our community" (Department for Communities & Local Government, 2010, p. 4). Apparently, many of our democratic institutions could not function in a transparent and inclusive way without those volunteers.

Secondly, there is political involvement in political parties and also lobbying, including taking action to write letter to MPs. At least four political parties in the UK promote volunteering opportunities on their websites promising "*a warm welcome from your local party*" (Labour Party, 2022) asking for volunteers to "*help elect Conservatives up and down the country*" (Conservative Party, 2022), "*helping to elect community champions*" (Liberal Democrats, 2022) and the Green Party (2022) stating that it is made up of 99% volunteers. This demonstrates how far the UK's political system fundamentally relies on volunteers.

2.2.5   Volunteering to Change the World

The report by United Nations Volunteers Programme (2021) uses the term campaigning to capture "*collective action*" to "*change the status quo*" (p. 19). It has many similarities with the type above, volunteering for democracy, but it is often undertaken outside the existing civic and political institutions. The campaign 'Insulate Britain' (2022) speaks of civil resistance to prevent a climate catastrophe, while 'Black Lives Matter' (2022) on its website states as the mission to "*eradicate white supremacy and build local power to intervene in violence inflicted on Black communities by the state and vigilantes*". As they are challenging the status quo, those volunteers are very likely to be self-organised and much less likely to get direct support from existing institutions, although there are increasingly opportunities to enable this. Campaigning and activist organisations such as Greenpeace call on volunteers to lobby at local level as, in their case, it "*has an impact on national and even global issues*" (Greenpeace, 2022).

2.2.6   Volunteering Abroad

Volunteering abroad goes back in time to the activities of missionaries in the eighteenth and nineteenth centuries and in the twentieth century to programmes such as the InterAmerican Student Project and Voluntary Services Overseas. More recently, a tourist industry has developed around providing volunteering opportunities abroad. Such volunteering has received criticism for its colonial past and attitudes, and for its hypocrisy, with Ivan Illich (1968) proclaiming "*to hell with good intentions*". Like all volunteering, it is neither inherently good nor bad, but in 'volunteering abroad', it is very important to ask questions relating to the purpose of volunteer involvement this chapter has raised, in particular with regards to perceptions of 'white saviourism'. Involving volunteers at great distance also brings an extra layer of responsibilities, to be further explored in Chapter Three.

2.2.7 'Not Being a Volunteer'

Not everyone who volunteers considers themselves a volunteer, nor does everyone who involves volunteers recognise this as volunteer involvement, nor themselves as involving volunteers and not everyone agrees on the basic definition of volunteering or the rationale for involving volunteers (Grotz et al., 2020). Because of this, a succession of observers have asked for a different word, to replace 'volunteer'. If people have a concept of volunteering, as perhaps being something for do-gooders or as not challenging current injustice, they may not want to identify themselves as volunteers, even if their activities match those included in this book's definition for volunteering. This emphasises that those who want to involve volunteers need to explain clearly what it is that they want to do, how and why. Informed volunteers can make informed choices regarding the way they want to volunteer. It is therefore not the word 'volunteer' that needs changing but those involving volunteers must explain clearly and transparently what volunteer involvement they seek. It is not acceptable to mask the purpose and meaning of volunteer involvement with opaque language and vague definition. Before we move to the next section on different models of volunteering, please consider the question in Exercise 2.3.

> **Exercise 2.3**
> In Exercise 1.4, we asked you who shouldn't be organising volunteering. Now, we'd like you to think about who should be responsible for organising volunteer involvement.

2.3   Two Models of Volunteer Involvement

The way volunteering is organised also varies greatly, not just because of the variety of rationales for volunteering but also because of the differences in activities undertaken. The volunteers of the Royal National Lifeboat Institution (RNLI) need to be exceptionally well-trained to deal with extremely dangerous situations and to be available on call to respond immediately when needed. Compare this to the volunteers who meet at the beach at a mutually agreed time or shared on social media, bring their own heavy duty plastic bags, and start collecting rubbish, without registering or being inducted. Having said that, an organisation might also be guiding volunteers who facilitate such beach-cleaning, keeping people safe (Surfers Against Sewage, 2022). The way volunteering is organised also depends on the way we conceptualise volunteering. To illustrate the effects of such different thinking, we introduce two distinctly different models of volunteer involvement: the transactional model and the participatory model.

The transactional model is mostly linked to the type 'philanthropic', 'service', 'volunteering for others' and appears to be favoured by the state. In NHS health and social care, the rationales which might be offered for involving volunteers within the transactional model relate to volunteers meeting a need by helping to deliver services. In its long-term plan, NHS England state: *"They* [volunteers] *enable staff to deliver high-quality care that goes above and beyond core services"* (NHS England, 2019). Volunteering within this model most commonly takes place within the large, volunteer involving organisations, which are run by paid staff.

The participatory model, on the other hand, is more akin to volunteer involvement for mutual aid, leisure, democracy and campaigning. It can be observed in associations run entirely by volunteers and relates to mutual benefits, as in self-help groups when people come together to address shared problems without professional support (Borkman, 1999). The two models are compared in Table 2.1.

Before we move to the next section on volunteer involvement and the state, we suggest you consider the question in Exercise 2.4 about the role the state should play.

Table 2.1 Two models of volunteer involvement

Transactional model	Participatory model
Volunteers are seen as unpaid labour	Volunteers are collaborators, members
Volunteers are passive, being recruited like staff, trained and directed	Volunteers are active, join, organise and participate
Mostly hierarchical	Less hierarchical
Aims, benefits are defined by organiser	Aims, benefits are defined by volunteers
Volunteers are directed	Volunteers direct

Exercise 2.4

What role should the state play in deciding why volunteering takes place, how it is organised and who is responsible for what?

2.4 Volunteer Involvement and the State

Wolch (1990) speaks of the possibility of a 'Shadow State' when discussing the relationship between the government and voluntary action, using the example of the Greater London Council as led by Ken Livingstone. With different administrations, these relationships change but are still important because government can significantly influence the environment for volunteer involvement. Furthermore, how willing volunteer involving organisations are to comply with government instruction can determine policy and practice. Government can make the conditions for volunteering easier through financial incentives but can also restrict it through regulations. The way governments do this is also important. Financial incentives can be distributed through local government funding volunteer centres but also through other institutions or programmes such as the National Citizen Service. Statutory regulations affecting volunteer involvement include the Lobbying Act, which has an impact on volunteering within the campaigning space. In 2014, the then Minister for Civil Society, Brooks Newmark, criticised charities for "*stray[ing] into the realm of politics*" by infamously exhorting them to "*stick to their knitting*" (Mason, 2014).

However, the influence of government can be overestimated. If we judge by numbers alone, none of the government incentives over the last decades, including the promotion of volunteering around the Olympics, have led to a long term, consistent increase in volunteering, nor has the relative neglect of volunteering in English policy over the last 10 years led to a significant overall reduction in volunteer numbers.

In the UK context since the early 2000s, national policies around volunteering are within devolved powers, so England, Wales, Scotland and Northern Ireland governments have different approaches. This has led to distinctly different developments regarding volunteer involvement in those nations (Hardill et al., 2022). At the time of writing this book, there is no dedicated minister or clear policy for volunteering in England, whereas in Scotland the 'Volunteering for All, national framework' aims to outline a "*coherent and compelling narrative for volunteering*" (Scottish Government, 2019, p. 4).

In England, the relationship between volunteering and the state has been changing over the last few decades with "*twists and turns, fits and starts, ups and downs, two steps forward and one step back*" (Zimmeck, 2010, p. 84) moving from the 'Mixed Economy of Welfare' via the 'Third Way' to the 'Big Society'.

Infrastructure organisations play an important role as intermediaries between volunteers, volunteer involving organisations and the state. Volunteer Scotland and Volunteer Now operate in Scotland and Northern Ireland respectively, whereas in England and Wales, umbrella organisations for the wider voluntary and community sector cover this function, the Wales Council for Voluntary Action (WCVA) and in England the National Council for Voluntary Organisations. Across the UK, they may collaborate with a range of local organisations dedicated to volunteering, such as volunteer centres and Councils for Voluntary Services. In Scotland, these are referred to as 'Third Sector Interfaces'. The past decade has seen many warnings about removal of local government funding leading to deconstruction of infrastructure in England. The Chief Executive of Volunteering England warned in 2012 that

"England's network of volunteer centres is at risk of "fragmentation" because of an average 12 per cent local authority funding cut" (Young, 2012).

But there are also other national bodies with departments dedicated to volunteering. Within England, in the health sector, Health Education England and NHS England, are likely to merge, both with a volunteer involvement function and, for sport, Sport England has a volunteering department. Add to this, the establishments delivering government programmes involving volunteering, either directly or through other infrastructure organisations and volunteer involving organisations, such as the National Citizen Service Trust, which has a mission to *"inspire generations of citizens through shared experiences that develop character and bridge social divides"* (National Citizen Service, 2022).

One of the possible confusions which then arise is to conflate understandings of the connection between the Voluntary Community and Social Enterprise sector and broader volunteer involvement. We have seen how volunteer involvement is not confined to charity and social enterprises but is found in every sector to some extent. Other evidence appears to show that not everyone who leads in the sector considers volunteer involvement to be central to what they do. Research published by New Philanthropy Capital showed only 51% of the charity chief executives saw volunteering as very important to achieving their mission, 10% thought volunteering was either 'slightly important' and 6% 'not important at all' (Murray et al., 2017, p. 35). They were also asked to identify the most important thing to help the charity sector increase its impact in society and only 4% of chief executives chose 'engaging users, stakeholders and volunteers' (p. 55).

This is an extremely complex landscape that differs across the nations of the UK and even locally, across England, with constant change in relationships between volunteer involvement and the state. In international comparisons, this landscape becomes even more complex in the face of socio-economic, political and cultural differences.

The next section will examine volunteer involvement and ideology. Before moving on, we suggest you consider the question in Exercise 2.5.

2.5   Volunteer Involvement and Ideology

Peter Beresford (2021) explains why we need to examine ideologies since *"we may not realise we are being influenced by them or even that we have them"* (p. 1). The way we have come to see the world underpins the way we volunteer, so that we will all bring our own ideologies to volunteering and those who involve volunteers will also bring their ideologies to how they structure volunteer involvement. This is particularly reflected in the rationales which organisations, groups and individuals offer for their volunteer involvement, permeating the way they organise it, what difference they want to make, how they judge this difference and how they see power as located through accountability.

In Sect. 2.2 of this chapter, we have described different ways people conceive volunteering, reflecting their own personal ideologies. In Sect. 2.3, we reflected on how an organisation's rationales and configurations influence how they organise volunteering in different models. And in Sect. 2.4, we have explained the role political ideology can play in the relationship between volunteer involvement and the state.

We now turn our attention to what this means in practice, how volunteer involvement practice is influenced by ideology, in particular how impact is assessed, where power is located and how accountability is regulated.

The difference volunteers make is often referred to as impact. How this is judged varies greatly and depends on what is measured, on where the difference is being made and for whom. Is it the difference volunteer involvement makes for people who are being helped or supported by volunteers, who are sometimes referred to as service users or beneficiaries. Measures can include assessments of what people learn from mentors or the practical help, such as respite care, they receive. Or is it the difference volunteering makes to the volunteer involving organisations? Volunteers can raise money for causes by taking part in sponsored events, or add perceived credibility to a group's position or message by adding their voice. Then there is the difference that volunteers make to the environment or broader communities, with river cleaning, festivities and improving access to culture such as museums and galleries. Finally, and increasingly receiving attention, the difference volunteering makes for the volunteer, ranging from personal well-being to the benefits of networking. Each of these can be measured in different ways, from simply counting the hours of volunteering taking place, money raised or saved, reputation of an organisation enhanced, reach and relevance broadened as well as changes to individual and public health.

The nature of volunteer involvement is determined by where the power for this is located. There are two main forms of volunteer involving organisations. About 20% of them are organisations with paid staff including commonly recognised charities and public bodies, such as an NHS Trust. Around 80% are those which are unincorporated and function as associations, being volunteer and member-led. The former is where transactional volunteering is more likely to be seen, where control rests with staff, as volunteers are likely involved specifically to one activity and allocated for pre-determined, utilitarian tasks. There is a clear distinction between the remits of volunteers and that of paid staff, including that volunteers don't need to fear financial loss or breach of contract from removing themselves from the activity. That is not to say that they wouldn't experience other loss from stepping away.

Compare this with volunteers coming together in associations without paid staff to run campaigns or leisure activities. Here control is mostly located with the individual. Having said that, even within seemingly non-hierarchical associations, power dynamics are likely to assert themselves. Particularly when coming together in associations, volunteers and the communities in which they are involved need to have or gain the power to affect change. This is recognised in the initiative Vision for Volunteering, which was recently launched by the National Association for Voluntary and Community Action (NAVCA), National Council for Voluntary Organisations (NCVO), Volunteering Matters, the Association of Volunteer Managers (AVM) and Sport England. On the website of the initiative, these organisations state that they are looking forward to a future *"where volunteering is understood as the community taking action, often enabled or supported by organisations, but not always driven or generated by them"* and in which *"communities are supported to experiment and innovate to develop their own solutions"* (Vision for Volunteering, 2022).

One other way to understand where power lies is to look at accountability and scrutiny. Many volunteer involving organisations have processes to monitor volunteers they involve, to ensure that they comply with policies, for example around ethical behaviour. There will also likely be processes to support the volunteer, including policies that ensure that volunteers have a way to address problems they face. However, this is not necessarily reciprocated as volunteers in those organisations might have little or no say in the running or scrutinising of the organisation.

This is different in groups that are predominantly volunteer run. Often, as for associations, these have statutes to regulate who does what and on what authority. However, while power appears shared and accountability to each other more regulated, problems with sharing power across the group are not uncommon.

Another element of organising volunteering, which reflects a truly participatory approach, is when people have a more collective purpose. Here, individuals in a community come together without setting up a regulatory framework but aim to share their strengths so as to jointly address a shared problem. In whichever way these groups are organised, they are often supported by some infrastructure, even if as simple as having a rota and regular communication which ensures that things are carried out effectively.

Two additional concepts of volunteers actively enabling organisations to be accountable to those they mean to benefit, are by first, playing a bridging role to reduce the distance between them (Dewi et al., 2019) and second, by volunteers taking ownership of broad public societal issues, such as crime prevention (Almond et al., 2015, p. 12), while invoking values of solidarity. Here, they can be seen as personally accountable for acting to generate social capital and acting as representatives of the broader public.

2.6   Summary and Conclusion

In this chapter, we explored the plurality of the ways volunteer involvement is conceived, encouraging you to consider different ways to understand volunteer involvement. In the section on volunteering history, we have explained how far back volunteer involvement goes. We then explained how people understand and conceptualise volunteering differently, organise it differently and how all this might be influenced by people's ideologies, meaning by the way they see the world.

We hope that this enables you to make your own judgements, not just about where in the complex landscape of volunteering your involvement activities are located and how you speak of it but also to assess what the various interests and views of each of the stakeholders are and how they affect your volunteer involvement practices.

References

Abel-Smith, B. (1964). *The hospitals 1800–1948*. Heinemann.

ACT UP London. (2022). *About*. Introduction on webpages of ACT UP London. https://actuplondon.wordpress.com/about/. Accessed 27 August 2022.

Almond, P., Bates, A., & Wilson, C. (2015). Circles of support and accountability: Criminal justice volunteers as the 'deliberative public.' *The British Journal of Community Justice, 13*(1), 25–40.

Aves, G. (1969). *The voluntary worker in social services: Report of a Committee Jointly set up by the Council for Social Service and the National Institute for Social Work Training*. Bedford Square Press and George Allen & Unwin.

Barker, P. (2016). *Philip Barker: 1866 and all that*. A blog on the website Inside the Games. https://www.insidethegames.biz/articles/1040094/philip-barker-1866-and-all-that. Accessed 27 August 2022.

Beresford, P. (2021). *Participatory ideology: From exclusion to involvement*. Policy Press.

Beveridge, L. (1948). *Voluntary action*. George Allen & Unwin.

Black Lives Matter. (2022). *About*. Page on the website of Black Lives Matter. https://blacklivesmatter.com/about/. Accessed 27 June 2022.

Borkman, T. (1999). *Understanding self-help/mutual aid: Experiential learning in the commons*. Rutgers University Press.

Bourdillon, A. F. C. (1945). *Voluntary social services: Their place in the modern state*. Methuen & Co Ltd.

Brewis, G., Russell, J., & Holdworth, C. (2010). *Bursting the bubble: Students, volunteering, and the community, full report*. Institute for Volunteering, Research and National Co-ordination Centre for Public Engagement.

Commission on the Future of the Voluntary Sector. (1996). *Meeting the challenge of change: Voluntary action into the 21st century*. NCVO.

Commission on the Future of Volunteering. (2008). *Report of the commission on the future of volunteering and manifesto for change*. Volunteering England.

Conservative Party. (2022). *Volunteer with us*. Landing page on the website. https://volunteer.conservatives.com/. Accessed 28 August 2022.

Covid-19 Mutual Aid UK. (2022a). Frequently asked questions. Page on the 117 website of COVID-19 Mutual Aid UK. https://covidmutualaid.org/faq/. Accessed 27 June 2022.

Covid-19 Mutual Aid UK. (2022b). *Homepage*. Page on the website of Covid-19 Mutual Aid UK. https://covidmutualaid.org. Accessed 27 June 2022.

Cowman K. (2018). *What life was like as a suffragette organizer*. Blog on the website of the British Academy. https://www.thebritishacademy.ac.uk/blog/what-life-was-suffragette-organiser/. Accessed 27 August 2022.

Davis Smith, J., Rochester, C., & Hedley, R. (1995). *An introduction to the voluntary sector*. Routledge.

Davis Smith, J. (2019). *100 years of NCVO and voluntary action: Idealists and realists*. Palgrave Macmillan.

Department for Communities and Local Government. (2010). *Volunteering for civic roles information for employers and employees*. Department for Communities and Local Government.

Dewi, M. K., Manochin, M., & Belal, A. (2019). Marching with the volunteers: Their role and impact on beneficiary accountability in an Indonesian NGO. *Accounting, Auditing & Accountability Journal, 32*(4), 1117–1145. https://doi.org/10.1108/AAAJ-10-2016-2727

Green Party. (2022). *Volunteer to get Greens elected*. Page on the website of the Green Party. https://campaigns.greenparty.org.uk/get-involved/. Accessed 28 August 2022.

Greenpeace. (2022). *Join the political lobbying network*. Page on the website of Greenpeace. https://www.greenpeace.org.uk/volunteering/join-the-political-lobbying-network/. Accessed 12 June 2022.

Grotz, J. (1992). *Das Blindenwesen in der Volksrepublik China; Staatlicher Anspruch und Realitat* (MA thesis). Marburg: Philipps-University.

Grotz, J., Ledgard, M., & Poland, F. (2020). *Patient and public involvement in health and social care: An introduction to theory and practice.* Imprint Springer Nature and Palgrave Macmillan.

Haldane, A. (2021). *The second invisible hand.* Local Trust Community Power Lecture. https://localtrust.org.uk/wp-content/uploads/2021/07/Andy-Haldane_Community-power-lecture_6-July.pdf. Accessed 28 August 2022.

Hardill, I., Grotz, J., & Crawford, L. (2022). *Mobilising voluntary action in the UK learning from the pandemic.* Policy Press.

Harris, B., Morris, A., Ascough, R. S., Chikoto, G. L., Elson, P. R., McLoughlin, J., Muukkonen, M., Pospíšilová, T., Roka, K., Smith, D. H., Soteri-Proctor, A., Tumanova, A. S., & Yu, P. J. (2016). History of associations and volunteering. In D. H. Smith, R. A. Stebbins, & J. Grotz (Eds.), *The Palgrave handbook of volunteering, civic participation, and nonprofit associations* (pp. 23–58). Palgrave Macmillan.

Insulate Britain. (2022). *Help support the Insulate Britain Campaign.* Homepage of insulatebritain.com. http://insulatebritain.com. Accessed 27 June 2022.

Illich, I. (1968). *Untitled talk delivered Saturday April 20 at St. Mary's Lake of the Woods Seminary in Niles (Chicago) Illinois, the talk is also referred to as 'to hell with good intentions'.* A text version of the speech was scanned from an original mimeograph distributed to Conference participants on the following day now available at The Conference on Interamerican Student Projects website. http://www.ciasp.ca/CIASPhistory/IllichCIASPspeech68.pdf. Accessed 26 June 2022.

Kropotkin, P. (1902). *Mutual aid: A factor of evolution.* Heineman.

Labour Party. (2022). *Volunteering FAQs.* Page on the website of The Labour Party. https://labour.org.uk/members/activist-area/budding-activists/volunteering-faqs/. Accessed 28 August 2022.

Liberal Democrats. (2022). *Become a volunteer today.* Page on the website of the Liberal Democrats. https://www.libdems.org.uk/volunteer. Accessed 28 August 2022.

Mason, R. (2014). *Charities should stick to knitting and keep out of politics, says MP.* The Guardian News Webpages 3 September 2014. https://www.theguardian.com/society/2014/sep/03/charities-knitting-politics-brook-newmark. Accessed 25 June 2022.

Murray, P., Shea, J., & Hoare, G. (2017). *Charities taking charge: Transforming to face a changing world*. New Philanthropy Capital. https://www.thinknpc. org/resource-hub/charities-taking-charge/. Accessed 27 August 2022.

National Citizen Service Trust. (2022). *About NCS Trust*. Page on the website of the National Citizen Service Trust. https://wearencs.com/about-ncs-trust. Accessed 28 August 2022.

National Council for Voluntary Organisations. (2018). *Impactful Volunteering, understanding the impact of volunteering on volunteers*. Research briefing on National Council for Voluntary Organisations webpages. https://www.ncvo. org.uk/images/documents/policy_and_research/Impactful-volunteering-und erstanding-the-impact-of-volunteering-on-volunteers.pdf. Accessed 25 June 2022.

NewStatesman Archive. (2021). *From the NS archive: Mr Chamberlain's fiasco 7 April 1917: A call for volunteers, but volunteering for what?* https://www.new statesman.com/2021/05/ns-archive-mr-chamberlain-s-fiasco. Accessed 27 August 2022. The authors are grateful to Dr Sandy MacDonald, University of Northampton for pointing out this report for the evidence collection of the project https://www.mvain4.uk

NHS England. (2019). *The NHS long term plan*. NHS England. https://www. longtermplan.nhs.uk/wp-content/uploads/2019/08/nhs-long-term-plan-ver sion-1.2.pdf. Accessed 27 August 2022.

Ockenden, N. (Ed.). (2007). *Volunteering works: Volunteering and social policy*. Institute for Volunteering Research and Volunteering England.

O'Hagan, M. (2001). *Stories from the edge*. Volunteer Development Agency, Northern Ireland. https://www.yumpu.com/en/document/read/52071572/ stories-from-the-edge-volunteer-now. Accessed 27 August 2022.

Rochester, C. (2013). *Rediscovering voluntary action*. Palgrave Macmillan.

Royal Society for the Protection of Birds. (2022). *Our history*. Page on the website of the Royal Society for the Protection of Birds. https://www.rspb. org.uk/about-the-rspb/about-us/our-history/. Accessed 28 June 2022.

Scottish Government. (2019). *Volunteering for all: Our national framework*. Scottish Government. https://www.gov.scot/publications/volunteering-nat ional-framework/. Accessed 27 June 2022.

Sport England. (2016). *Volunteering in an active nation*. Sport England. https://sportengland-production-files.s3.eu-west-2.amazonaws.com/s3fs- public/2020-01/volunteering-in-an-active-nation-final.pdf?VersionId=LU3 cqHb9FZvVWi3rye.b.HNIe5UM9wOX. Accessed 26 June 2022.

Stebbins, R., & Graham, M. (Eds.). (2004). *Volunteering as leisure/leisure as volunteering: An International Assessment*. CABI Publishing.

Surfers Against Sewage. (2022). *Organise your million mile clean*. Page on the website of Surfers Against Sewage. https://www.sas.org.uk/our-work/beach-cleans/organise-beach-clean. Accessed 26 June 2022.

United Nations General Assembly. (2001). *UNGA Resolution 56/38: Recommendations on support for volunteering*. Page on website of UN Volunteers. https://www.unv.org/publications/unga-resolution-5638-recommendations-support-volunteering. Accessed 28 June 2022.

United Nations Volunteers (UNV) Programme. (2021). *2022 state of the world's volunteerism report. Building equal and inclusive societies*. United Nations Volunteers (UNV) programme.

Vision for Volunteering. (2020). How does volunteering need to adapt by 2032? Landing page on the website of the Vision for Volunteering. https://www.visionforvolunteering.org.uk. Accessed 27 August 2022.

Volans, I. (2010). *Die Turnhalle: Britains first gymnasium*. Page on the website SportingLandmarks.co.uk. https://sportinglandmarks.co.uk/die-turnhalle-britains-first-gymnasium/. Accessed 27 August 2022.

Wolch, J. (1990). *The shadow state: Government and voluntary sector in transition*. The Foundation Centre.

Wolfenden Committee. (1978). *The future of voluntary organisations*. Croom Helm.

Young, N. M. (2012). *Volunteer centre network 'will fragment' under council cuts*. Page on Civil Society News website. https://www.civilsociety.co.uk/news/volunteer-centre-network--will-fragment--under-council-cuts.html. Accessed 27 August 2022.

Zimmeck, M. (2010). Government and volunteering: Towards a history of policy and practice. In C. Rochester, E. P. Angela, & S. Howlett, with M. Zimmeck (Eds.), *Volunteering and society in the 21st century* (pp. 84–102). Palgrave Macmillan.

3

Critical Perspectives and Potential Negative Impacts

Abstract Chapter Three first explores critical perspectives on volunteer involvement and the effects of misconduct, including 'transgression'. It then discusses the negative impacts of volunteering and examines consequences of the 'benefit fallacy'. It encourages the reader to use five 'Exercises' to reflect on critical perspectives they have encountered and on examples of misconduct or negative impacts in their own experience.

Keywords Misconduct · Negative impacts · Benefit fallacy

Volunteer involvement is not always an inherently good thing. Before we start this chapter, please reflect on your own views of others, who view and speak of volunteer involvement negatively by considering the questions in Exercise 3.1.

© The Author(s), under exclusive license to Springer Nature Switzerland AG 2022
J. Grotz and R. Leonard, *Volunteer Involvement*,
https://doi.org/10.1007/978-3-031-19221-0_3

Exercise 3.1

Think of examples of people speaking negatively about volunteering. What are they saying and what do you think about their views?

3.1   Criticism

Over decades, many volunteer involving organisations and others with an interest, such as politicians, have promoted volunteering with an angelic image and a narrative of volunteers as 'saints' and 'heroes', whose involvement offers social, economic and cultural value. Promoting the virtues of volunteer involvement is pervasive and entrenched in the UK, not just in the media but also in evaluating many programmes. Recent examples of promoting such virtues in the media range from reports of support for Ukranian refugees and the Commonwealth Games, to organising foodbanks, and describing how volunteers respond to current opportunities and crises.

At the same time, critical views have been sidelined and even in tasks such as 'good practice development', organisations appear to mostly look for ways to measure success and identify evidence to the contrary only as barriers to success. This narrative is supported by an impressive body of evidence pointing out the benefits of volunteering, broadly categorising them as benefits to the volunteers, benefits to the volunteer involving organisations, and benefits to the wider community.

Based on this narrative, it is unsurprising that policymakers have consistently seen volunteering as a great force for good. Before the UK elections in 2010, the Conservative Party, then in coalition government declared that:

> ...volunteers are the beating heart of Britain's civil society, an indispensable resource for the voluntary sector and in many public services. Volunteering generates social capital—building the networks that turn mere places into communities. In economic terms, the value of volunteering can be measured in billions of pounds, but its true worth is

beyond price. Without volunteers much of what we take for granted in our national life would grind to a halt. (Conservative Party, 2008, p. 20)

Ed Miliband, the then Opposition Leader in his speech on 'Responsibility in 21st Century Britain', London 13 June 2011, also referred to volunteers as the *"unsung heroes who make such a difference to the lives of others"* (Miliband, 2011).

Today, governments and others still seek to utilise the benefits of volunteering. The report to the government by MP Danny Kruger 'Levelling up our communities: proposals for a new social covenant' (2020) recommends developing solutions to match the supply of citizens to the demand of time that could drive more and better volunteering, while the Prime Minister Boris Johnson called on 14 December 2021 *"for volunteers to join our national mission to get jabs in arms. We need tens of thousands of people to help out—everyone from trained vaccinators to stewards"* (Johnson, 2021). Multiple initiatives such as the National Citizen Service (NCS), a programme for 16 and 17 year olds, which included volunteering in a wider range of activities, and #IWill which encouraged anyone under 25 years old to contribute to society by campaigning, volunteering or fundraising, exist to encourage involvement for young people and others in volunteering. Such initiatives appeared to be based on the explicit assumption that volunteering is beneficial and largely unproblematic.

However, as we shall see in this chapter, the accounts provided by volunteers do not seem to be as supportive and uncritical, when compared to what volunteer involving organisations focus on and there are other, often unheard, critical voices. People are asking questions that seriously challenge our assumptions.

- Is volunteering really a force for good or does it help sustain injustices?
- Does it help to make young people more employable or does it exploit them and threaten other people's jobs?
- Is volunteering a privilege or a duty?
- Are volunteer involving organisations up to the job or do they need regulations like those which govern fundraising?

* Are those who call on volunteers in emergencies well enough prepared to involve them?

Such questions raise important moral and ethical issues. They directly challenge those who would leave unrecorded and unaddressed the potentially negative impacts of volunteering, which contradict the narrative of benefits, trying to avoid damage to organisations' images and priorities. We must clearly acknowledge that critical views of volunteer involvement are not always welcome. Those who put these views forward might be criticised for simply stating evidence. This chapter should act as a general warning to practitioners.

We will first explore critical perspectives on volunteering, including views of volunteering as unpaid labour or as a reserve force, the challenge of 'NIMBYism' and also areas such as volunteer tourism where volunteering might be seen to display a colonial legacy and so to perpetuate the very issues it ostensibly wants to address. We will then look at misconduct and the many other aspects which may go wrong in volunteer involvement, arranging them in the same ways benefits are usually arranged, by looking at negative impacts on volunteers, volunteer involving organisations and the wider community. The end of the chapter will discuss the consequences of not adequately recognising critical views and dangers associated with a bias towards reporting benefits, in a section on the 'benefit fallacy'.

Before we move on to explore negative views of others, to help you locate your own views, please consider the question in Exercise 3.2 reflecting on when you personally might view volunteering as negative, whether you are a volunteer or paid staff.

Exercise 3.2

Consider why paid staff might see involving volunteers in their own organisation as negative.

3.1.1 Volunteers as Unpaid Labour

A report on volunteering in the NHS by the Institute for Volunteering Research and the National Association of Volunteer Service Managers asserts the following:

> Concern about job substitution was stronger in trusts where volunteers were given administrative duties to perform. Volunteering tended to receive most support from paid staff when volunteers were current or former service users. (Teasdale, 2008a, p. 5)

Especially during times of austerity and worries regarding job security, there can be concerns that organisations make what are perceived to be money-saving decisions by substituting volunteers for paid staff. Historically, the most vocal opponents of volunteering as unpaid labour have probably been the trade unions. To address these challenges, the Trades Union Congress (TUC) and Volunteering England developed a Charter in 2009 to strengthen the relationship between paid staff and volunteers in any organisation (Trades Union Congress, 2009).

However, nearly a decade later Unison's report on Police Support Volunteers 'Crossing the Line', still explores concerns that volunteers are being used to backfill police staff roles citing that the number of Police Support Volunteers (PSVs) increased by nearly 1,000 between 2014 and 2017 while over the same time, the number of paid police staff jobs was cut by over 1,500.

> Volunteering can be valuable to police forces, rewarding for the PSVs, and a valuable bridge between a community and their police force, but questions need to be asked when volunteering spills over into areas that were previously the preserve of directly employed, highly trained, vetted, and skilled police employees. We have to ask whether communities and the volunteers themselves are being put at risk, unsustainable strategies being promoted, and communities short-changed. (Unison, 2018a, p. 7)

The Unison General Secretary at the time Dave Prentis, said: "*The concern is they're being taken on partly to compensate for the loss of tens of thousands of paid police staff and officers as a result of government cuts*" (Unison, 2018b).

Even if not viewed as a direct threat to employment, volunteers might be seen by staff as outsiders interfering or as a management tool to report on staff (Teasdale, 2008a, 2008b). Likewise volunteers feel that in such circumstances, they cannot have a positive volunteering experience (McGarvey et al., 2020, p. 32).

Further dimensions of this are unpaid internships and placements as well as inviting people to become involved in the design and direction of services, under the guise of 'engagement', especially if it is in programmes that return income to the volunteer involving organisation. Criticism of unpaid commercial internship as exploitative and only open to the more privileged has been joined by criticism of charities as following a similar path.

> Charities are asking interns to work 252 hours unpaid. That's a scandal…Internships are not volunteering opportunities and charities do not have a universal right to unpaid talent. (Ward, 2017)

In the name of 'participation', volunteers are also often invited to take part in consultations on policy and in research, for example in patient and public involvement.

> [Patient and Public Involvement] PPI is a form of volunteering; indeed, it is many forms of volunteering. It is therefore relevant and important for us to apply wider lessons from good practice in involving volunteers to inform the good practice in PPI. (Grotz et al., 2020, p. 16)

However, this appears often undertaken without fully considering the ethics of such involvement and, in particular, how important good volunteering experiences are, including volunteers understanding how they are making a difference. As in other forms of volunteer involvement, consulting is infrequently informed by enough evidence and fails to address persistent inequalities. Madden and Speed (2017) speak of

'Zombies and Unicorns' when they discuss the range of expectations from stakeholders like funders, health professionals and, of course, the volunteers and suggest that:

> This zombie/unicorn hybrid creates [Patient and Public Involvement] PPI as a form of busywork in which the politics of social movements are entirely displaced by technocratic discourses of managerialism.

3.1.2 Volunteers as a Reserve Force in Emergencies

The volunteering responses to the 2020–2022 COVID-19 pandemic are a clear expression of our humanity but they also laid bare an error that has been repeated by governments over and over again, conflating the willingness of people to help in an emergency with the capacity to deploy those volunteers in a coordinated response.

On the one hand, volunteers are quickly found but then are not asked to do anything, while on the other hand, the spontaneous volunteers, who organise themselves, are viewed suspiciously as not being 'professionals' or not following appropriate regulations. As we saw in Chapter Two, examples of these attitudes and practices go back over centuries and are repeated over and over again, which is fully recognised in available evidence.

> Volunteering in emergencies, crises, and disasters nearly always occurs, despite being ignored by some professional emergency managers and government officials. Unfortunately, when crisis/disaster plans are written up to try to mitigate and respond to future incidents, the untrained disaster volunteer and the emergent process of which she/he is a part, is usually not included explicitly among the explicit dimensions of the plan. (Aguirre et al., 2016, p. 311)

COVID-19 Mutual Aid Groups have been recognised and credited with providing key responses but it is also clear that they encountered practical

and other obstacles. Some of these obstacles might be linked to contra-
dictions arising from treating volunteers as a reserve army, which may be
at odds with the effectiveness of collaborating in a collectivist community
way (Tiratelli & Kaye, 2020, p. 24).

3.1.3 Volunteering for 'Not in My Back Yard' Campaigns

Volunteering is seen as a vital component in achieving 'stronger and
safer' communities, such as through 'neighbourhood watch' groups.
Putnam (2000) speaks of the value of social capital which enables better
connected communities to achieve outcomes more effectively. While
local campaigning is sometimes heralded as a return of power to the
community, it is also associated with NIMBYism, a pejorative term
referring to a 'not in my backyard' attitude.

In contradiction to the belief that volunteering will make the whole
community stronger and safer, there is evidence that it can be divisive
and exclusive. Aldrich and Crook offer the example of how when siting
Trailers in Post-Katrina New Orleans, civil society worked simultane-
ously to bring citizens together while mobilising them against the threat
of trailer parks in their backyards (Aldrich & Crook, 2008).

3.1.4 Volunteering as Antiquated and Colonial

Two contexts might be looked at here. Firstly, the idea of volunteer
involvement as patronising and paternalistic charity rather than empowering communities, and secondly volunteer tourism. Peter Beresford
(2016) describes how welfare policies in the UK may perpetuate concepts
such as the 'deserving poor'. Volunteering can be seen to do the same,
by preserving the system rather than challenging it. Of course, volunteer involvement takes place around the globe and in many cultures,
with a variety of concepts and with other underlying purposes (United
Nations Volunteers Programme, 2021). Exploring them and reflecting
on whether or not different forms of volunteer involvement empower

rather than patronise might be beneficial for a more comprehensive understanding of volunteer involvement.

Criticisms have also been and continue to be raised in the context of volunteering in international development.

> I have become known for my increasing opposition to the presence of any and all North American 'dogooders' in Latin America. (Illich, 1968, p. 3)

Today, this criticism extends to the impact of volunteer tourism on the host communities (Smith & Holmes, 2009). Here is a vivid more recent observation:

> 'There are few things more cringeworthy than watching 20 British schoolgirls trying to build a well under the scalding Nepalese heat,' one Durham University student wrote about her trip to an orphanage. Villagers, wary of offending their visitors, say nothing. (May 2018 cited in Rosenberg, 2018)

Such critical views are not hidden but they do not seem to feature in the broader discourse of the promotion of volunteer involvement.

3.2   Misconduct

Misconduct is defined as a behaviour not conforming to prevailing standards or laws. It is a recognised phenomenon when involving people, volunteers as well as staff. It ranges from minor issues such as persistently bad timekeeping, taking on tasks which go beyond the agreed remit, to much more serious issues such as failure to respect clients' or customers' confidentiality, dignity, independence and individuality, breach of health and safety regulations or agreements, misuse of the organisation's equipment or facilities, theft, discrimination on grounds of disability, race, gender and abuse or other offensive behaviour, including arriving for the activity under the influence of alcohol or drugs, or other substance abuse.

Misconduct in volunteer involvement is well-known with some guidance provided by national umbrella organisations, such as the National Council for Voluntary Organisations (no date) in England and Volunteer Now (2022) in Northern Ireland.

Below we will briefly discuss misconduct by volunteers, by volunteer involving organisations and misconduct through transgression. Before we do, we would like to encourage you to reflect on examples of misconduct in volunteer involvement you have encountered. See Exercise 3.3.

Exercise 3.3

Think of examples of misconduct in volunteer involvement you have personally encountered rather than heard of.

3.2.1 Misconduct of Volunteers

Misconduct of volunteers is well recognised and dealt with in many volunteer involving organisations. According to a report by the Institute for Volunteering Research, 74% of the 547 organisations they surveyed had procedures for dealing with problems involving volunteers (Institute for Volunteering Research, 1998). Yet, while many organisations have adopted a workplace model for their involvement of volunteers and deal with problems accordingly (Rochester et al.,. 2010, p. 150), the same organisations involving volunteers are advised strictly, not to enter into any contractual agreement with volunteers as they need to keep the status of volunteers and that of paid staff explicitly different. This may cause them a problem, as Volunteering England pointed out, because volunteers are "*under no obligation to stay*" (Volunteering England, 2009, p. 5). The interim report of the Volunteer Rights Inquiry quotes respondents:

> "When facing any formal inquiry about the volunteering they have undertaken" this "is the most difficult if volunteers chose to resign rather than engage with any inquiry. (Volunteer Rights Inquiry, 2010, p. 12)

However, this is not exclusive to volunteer involving organisations with a 'workplace model', even community-led mutual aid groups face such difficulties as was demonstrated in Tiratelli and Kaye's research:

> Despite their successes, the Mutual Aid groups that we have spoken to for this research have encountered a range of challenges, from managing the conduct and morale of volunteers, to working out how best to structure themselves. (2020, p. 21)

Misconduct can take dramatic and extremely distressing forms which require safeguarding mechanisms, as evidenced in the report to the Secretary of State for Health regarding the lessons learnt from NHS investigations into matters relating to Jimmy Savile (Lampard & Marsden, 2015). These have shown that there is a shared responsibility to protect everyone and that this is a well-established concept in volunteer involvement.

> ....repeating such abuses can only be avoided if all volunteer involving organisations can refer to and act on a clear shared understanding. It requires repeated reinforcement of messages, awareness-raising and training, as well as regular ongoing testing of the effectiveness and relevance of safeguarding arrangements. (Grotz et al., 2020)

Volunteer involving organisations use a range of measures, including requesting background checks like from Disclosure and Barring Service (DBS) in England or Protecting Vulnerable Groups (PVG) scheme in Scotland, to make sure that people with a history of abuse cannot volunteer in specific activities.

3.2.2 Misconduct by Volunteer Involving Organisations

However, what happens when there is misconduct displayed not by the volunteers but by the organisation for which they volunteer? In 2008, John Stoker presented his report of a review of the York Citizens Advice Bureau. He had found that *"Breaches of the procedures were pervasive and serious and involved detriment and unfairness"* (Stoker, 2008, p. 13).

Volunteers affected had no mechanism to challenge this, so they chose a course of action reminiscent of an industrial dispute, they walked out. This case confirmed not only that conflict between volunteers and volunteer involving organisations exist but highlighted the fact that despite some organisations having policies in place, volunteering, such as at Citizens Advice, is largely unregulated in the UK without legal mechanism to deal with conflict.

Policy documents such as the Report of the Commission on the Future of Volunteering and Manifesto for Change seem to deal with this by recommending regulation:

> regulatory bodies, such as the Healthcare Commission, the Commission for Social Care Inspection and Ofsted should include as part of their regular inspections an assessment of how organisations involve, support and manage volunteers in order to provide high quality and user sensitive services. (Commission on the Future of Volunteering, 2008, p. 32)

However, Grotz and Locke (2022) point out that unlike in fundraising, no such regulation has been introduced and discuss the possible reasons for this comparing 'volunteers and the law' and 'volunteer rights'. The interim report of the Volunteer Rights Inquiry adds a whole list of areas of misconduct in other volunteer involving organisations, reported by volunteers, ranging from bullying and intimidation to breaches of trust. What advice is given to volunteers when they are the subject of misconduct? Currently, the answer is still the same as this one in 2009, leave.

> Ultimately, if you do have a negative volunteering experience, try to remember that this is the exception rather than the rule, and that many people view their volunteering in a positive light. If the organisation you volunteer with is unable to provide a suitable solution, remember that you are under no obligation to stay and that there are numerous organisations, ranging from charities, voluntary organisations, community groups and statutory agencies, such as hospitals, schools or museums, which are actively seeking volunteers and would welcome an addition to their volunteering team. (Volunteering England, 2009, p. 5)

However, the interim report of the Volunteer Rights Inquiry also highlights consequences for volunteers who cannot or do not want to leave if a situation cannot be resolved or who are seeking redress. Leaving these volunteers without the right "*to have an organisation follow proper investigative procedures*" (Volunteering England, 2010, p. 2) is relevant to any initiatives reducing the element of free will in volunteering activities. This includes any volunteering associated with welfare payments, especially 'back to work' programmes, the National Citizen Service, and 'compulsory' elements in education courses. If the element of choice is impeded to such an extent that stopping a volunteering activity would have negative consequences, such as failing a course, the danger of further negative consequences increases and we must question whether the activity still falls within the definition of volunteering. It does also affect other instances where individuals, particularly vulnerable individuals, might require protection from misconduct or from pressure to stay in a volunteering position as in placements or internships. Despite this evidence, the National Council for Voluntary Organisations (2014) reporting on outcomes of the Volunteer Rights Enquiry recommended self-regulation rather than regulation to ensure compliance and redress.

3.2.3 Misconduct as Transgression

Some voluntary groups are set up with purposes or for activities which do not conform with prevailing standards or laws while other groups might choose a course of action which does not conform with, or even deliberately or otherwise transgresses, prevailing standards or laws to pursue particular objectives. In his study of 'deviant' non-profit groups, Smith (2019) offers examples ranging from 'delinquent gangs' and 'swinger clubs' to 'cults' and 'revolutionary groups'. In transgressive volunteer involvement both the potentially contentious purpose of the volunteer involvement and also how volunteer activities actually break norms or even laws characterise the activity. An example was the Insulate Britain activists who the judge said they had "inspired me personally" while recognising his own role to apply the law (Thomas, 2022).

It is of course very difficult to capture transgression, as norms and laws change or vary in other countries. So, what was once acceptable in Victorian London, might be no longer and could even be illegal today, or what is acceptable now might then have caused outrage or led to imprisonment. Something encouraged and promoted in Britain today, might still be illegal in another country. One person's terrorist is another one's freedom fighter, one's campaigner for the unborn life is another one's bigot, and one's internet funny guys are another's stalkers. But all might still be volunteering. Who decides and on what criteria? And of course transgressive volunteer involvement can have a purpose all by itself.

In light of this discussion and before we move to negative impacts of volunteering, please ask yourself the question in Exercise 3.4, considering examples of volunteering that you feel should not be allowed.

Exercise 3.4

What volunteering should not be allowed?

3.3 Negative Impacts

In this section, we will explore evidence that has been emerging for at least a decade suggesting that volunteering might not always be of benefit and sometimes might, unintentionally or intentionally, be harmful (Grotz, 2010, 2011). Like in other sections, we will be looking first at the impact on volunteers, then on volunteer involving organisations and finally at the negative impacts on the wider community. But before we go on, we would like you to consider the question in Exercise 3.5, thinking of examples when things went wrong in volunteer involvement and what the consequences of this were.

3.3.1 Negative Impact of Volunteering on Volunteers

Further to the negative impacts caused by misconduct of volunteers and volunteer involving organisations outlined above, there are other possible negative impacts on volunteers. In direct contradiction to the view that volunteering is a means of gaining confidence and self-esteem, the potential for emotional harm from volunteering was identified during the Volunteer Rights Inquiry. Witnesses to the Inquiry reported how their volunteering experience left them *"physically and mentally in pieces"* as they had been *"continually harassed, bullied, and worn down"* (Volunteering England, 2010, p. 7). Also directly contradicting the view that volunteering leads to better physical and mental health are studies which provide medical evidence of harm, such as in post-traumatic stress in volunteer fire fighters (Bryant & Harvey, 1996) and burnout in AIDS volunteers (Ross et al., 1999). We must ask whether those negative impacts are linked to the activity and the way it is undertaken rather than it being voluntary as it is likely that paid fire fighters will also experience post-traumatic stress (Thoits & Hewitt, 2001). We must equally ask whether volunteers who do not have specialist professional training might be at higher risk (Twigg & Mosel, 2017, p. 451).

Volunteering both through organisations and volunteering as individuals, not through groups, can even be fatal. While the RNLI reports that its volunteers have saved 139,000 lives at sea since 1824, 778 of its volunteers and crew are commemorated on the RNLI Memorial who have lost their own lives trying to save others (Grotz, 2011). As the next example of a fatality during volunteering not organised by a group suggests, we might ask whether volunteers are more likely to put themselves in dangerous situations, in dangerous waters. In the Postman's Park in London, plaques commemorate the self-sacrifice of people who died trying to save others. One of these plaques reads:

> Herbert Maconoghu, schoolboy from Wimbledon aged 13, his parents absent in India, lost his life in vainly trying to rescue his two school fellows who were drowned at Glovers Pool, Croyde, North Devon, August 28 1882. (Grotz, 2011)

This evidence of negative impact on individual volunteers clearly contradicts the assumption that volunteering is exclusively beneficial. Additionally, as a corollary of the qualification that we don't know whether or not these negative impacts might be linked to the activity rather than the fact that it is undertaken voluntarily, we must also apply this to evaluating the potential benefits of volunteering.

3.3.2 Negative Impact of Volunteering on Volunteer Involving Organisations

The negative impacts volunteering can have on volunteer involving organisations are exemplified by the fact that many such organisations have problem solving policies in place to address concerns regarding volunteers' behaviours and actions. An article in Volunteering England's good practice bank identified some of the circumstances under which volunteers may be disciplined including theft and poor behaviour. The financial impact of theft is obvious yet the impact on the service users of organisations, as in failing to respect clients or customers' confidentiality, dignity and independence can be much more subtle. Involvement of volunteers also requires some organisations to carefully consider their industrial relations as paid staff could feel threatened by an increased involvement of volunteers. This need for clarity within organisations is strongly expressed in the principles of volunteering endorsed by Greater London Volunteering: "*Like-for-like substitution of volunteers for paid staff is as unacceptable as redundant staff being replaced by new staff in the same role*" (Greater London Volunteering, 2010).

When volunteer involving organisations assess whether their investment in volunteer involvement is economically viable, they find that especially during the initial years of setting up volunteering offers, return from investment might be negative, meaning it might be cheaper to employ people or not pursue the activity at all.

Again, the evidence of potentially negative impacts on volunteer involving organisations either through actions of volunteers, wasted resources or the need to manage industrial relations directly contradicts the view that volunteering is exclusively beneficial for volunteer involving organisations.

3.3.3 Negative Impact of Volunteering on Beneficiaries and the Wider Community

Volunteering is commonly linked to the creation of social capital. Yet, Putnam (2000) points out that social capital itself is not intrinsically beneficial but can be directed to malevolent and antisocial purposes. He quotes the grand wizard of the Royal Knights of the Ku Klux Klan as saying: "*We want to be involved in the community*" (p. 22). Clearly there are volunteer run organisations in the UK which promote sectarianist or extremist views and either have or seek close community links.

When considering the impact of volunteering in campaigns, we should recognise that a campaign expressing one view may result in a counter-campaign expressing an opposite view and perceiving outcomes in many different ways. Some of the complexity of issues here can be illustrated by the activities of the British Disabled Angling Association (2021) which "*aims to provide new inclusive environments for angling, and to empower disabled people with an interest in angling and providing inclusive environments reduce dependency on others, empower individuals*" for which volunteers have an "*essential role in the charities operations*". While the British Disabled Angling Association's aims might generally be seen as benign, some angling saboteurs in the UK stated that: "*Angling is the Cruellest [activity] and Must Be Banned Now—there are No Arguments to defend the angling scum and their cruelty*" and have threatened action against all anglers, including disabled anglers (http://www.anti-angling-sabs.co.uk/, no longer available, cited in Grotz, 2009, p. 6). How deep such divisions can be and how dangerous the resulting actions of volunteers can be observed in the currently re-ignited *pro-life versus pro-choice* debate, following recent rulings in the USA.

Furthermore, while volunteering is credited for its economic contribution to communities, '*Valuable practical services ... are accomplished in the community that can reduce municipal costs and taxes or can improve municipal efficiency*' (Smith, 2000, p. 203), it is difficult to assess the municipal cost of volunteering, which may be caused unintentionally or intentionally. However, we can ask what the clean-up and policing costs of large-scale street carnivals are. Volunteering England's campaign, '*Volunteering is freely given but not cost free*', identified the need for funding relating to promotion, diversity, management and infrastructure within volunteering yet did not appear to identify direct municipal costs.

The above examples of negative impacts like being part of community conflict and economic costs, directly contradict the view that volunteering is solely beneficial for the wider community.

3.3.4 The Benefit Fallacy

Why, despite critical views, misconduct and clear evidence of non-beneficial effects of volunteering, unintentional and intentional, unrecognised or fully recognised, does there appear to have been so few attempts to include these in the wider discussion of volunteering? The reason may of course be found in attempts to sanitise the image of volunteering but it also lies in its very definition.

As we saw in Chapter One, a common definition of volunteering, by 2001, contained three key components: being uncoerced, unpaid and of benefit (United Nations General Assembly, 2001). When volunteering is by definition 'of benefit', there can be a bias in speaking only of volunteering which is seen to be of benefit, because otherwise it is not seen as volunteering. McCord (2003) also suggests that "*Evidence about adverse effects from social programs is hard to find in part because of a strong bias against reporting adverse effects of social programs. Authors of studies that fail to produce evidence of beneficial outcomes sometimes do not bother to submit their reports for publication*" (p. 26).

This could help to explain the mountain of evidence pointing towards benefits and the comparatively minimal exploration of negative impacts. The real potential for damage, however, is the resulting false assumption from its older definition, that ALL volunteering is of benefit. The unshakeable association, by definition, of volunteering and benefit has led to what appears to be failure to understand aspects of volunteering which few would associate with benefits, yet which fall into a definition of unpaid, uncoerced and of disputed or little benefit to others. This raises questions as to what the criteria are according to which the government decides whether or not an unpaid and uncoerced activity has "*added social value*" in voluntary service, civic service or civilian service (Commission of the European Communities, 2004, p. 5).

Some commentators like Smith (2008) call for awareness of the 'dark side' of the non-profit sector. Rochester characterises "*the arena of voluntary action as wide sprawling and untidy*" (Rochester et al., 2010, p. 243) yet still having boundaries. It appears that the boundaries around misconduct still need to be drawn. That is why at the beginning of this book, we suggested you to consider what volunteering is.

In 2002, the then Home Secretary David Blunkett had the National Coalition of Anti-Deportation Campaigns (NCADC) investigated and sought to stop it receiving a grant from the Big Lottery Fund as it was seen to help fight deportations, a topic recently reappearing. We must ask, are NCADC volunteers who are helping people facing deportation with how to launch and run anti-deportation campaigns part of what politicians describe as Britain's 'beating heart'? Is it just those volunteers who are doing what they are officially told, carrying out approved activities, who are the 'beating heart'? If those, such as the NCADC volunteers who may be acting against guidance are not viewed as volunteers, then David Blunkett's intervention exemplifies the relevance of this non-compliant form of volunteering to current policy, but not as automatically approved by policies. Alongside, a clear commitment to invest public funds in volunteering there needs to be transparency regarding what is included in the concept and importantly, what is not, and why not.

To simply assume that all volunteering is whatever is supported and is therefore of benefit, and alternatively that everything else is not volunteering is at the core of the 'benefit fallacy'. Whatever is not considered volunteering is not being measured and the negative effects of activities considered volunteering are not being made visible and therefore not fully understood.

3.4   Summary and Conclusion

In this chapter, we have reflected on diversity. We explored some of the negative views of volunteering as unpaid labour, as an emergency 'army', the effects of NIMBYism and antiquated and paternalistic or colonial views. We have described some examples of misconduct and have highlighted an extensive data- and cognitive-gap between the artificially created mountain of evidence asserting the benefits of volunteering alongside the comparatively minimal exploration of negative impacts. While it is likely that, as the available evidence suggests, benefits of volunteering far outweigh negative impacts, it is inconceivable that an activity in which millions of people participate every day is without negative impacts. Not answering difficult questions and a lack of recognition of negative views and negative impacts may result in serious consequences.

* Not listening to alternative accounts and not recognising other knowledges, may lead to less involvement with communities who hold different views or values.
* Ignoring negative impacts may put volunteers at risk by not exploring the dangers of volunteering.
* Distorting evidence with a bias on benefits may lead to errors in policymaking, in particular by an endeavour to maximise the involvement of volunteers without addressing risks.
* Withholding evidence of the negative aspects of volunteering may lead to a backlash in the future, if people feel misinformed.

If the desire to promote volunteering leads to a lack of clarity and transparency regarding all the aspects volunteer involvement entails, then, the longer such lack of clarity prevails, the greater any ultimate backlash could be. It seems therefore imperative to acknowledge and respond to negative views of volunteering, recognise the 'benefit fallacy' and to ensure that any future debate will include questions regarding both the benefits and negative impacts of volunteering. This more inclusive approach, helping to identify evidence that volunteering can also kill or harm and make the lives of volunteers and others a misery, might also strengthen any evidence that volunteering can save and prolong lives, empower those without power and lead to better quality of life.

References

Aguirre, B. E., Macias-Medrano, J., Batista-Silva, J. L., Chikoto, G. L., Jett, Q. R., & Jones-Lungo, K. (2016). Spontaneous volunteering in emergencies. In D. H. Smith, R. A. Stebbins, & J. Grotz (Eds.), *The Palgrave handbook of volunteering, civic participation, and nonprofit associations* (Vol. 1, pp. 311–329). Palgrave Macmillan.

Aldrich, D. P., & Crook, K. (2008). Strong civil society as a double-edged sword: Siting trailers in post-Katrina New Orleans. *Political Research Quarterly, 61*(3), 379–389.

Beresford, P. (2016). *All our welfare: Toward a participatory social policy*. Bristol: Policy Press.

British Disabled Angling Association. (2021). *Report of the trustees and unaudited financial statements for the year ended 30 June 2021*. British Disabled Angling Association.

Bryant, R. A., & Harvey, A. G. (1996). Posttraumatic stress reactions in volunteer fire fighters. *Journal of Traumatic Stress, 9*(1), 51–62.

Commission of the European Communities. (2004). *SEC(2004) 628 commission staff working paper—Analysis of the replies of the Member States of the European Union and the acceding countries to the Commission questionnaire on voluntary activities of young people*. Commission of the European Communities. http://ec.europa.eu/youth/archive/whitepaper/post-launch/sec(2004)628_en.pdf. Accessed 16 March 2010.

Commission on the Future of Volunteering. (2008). *Report of the commission on the future of volunteering and manifesto for change.* Volunteering England.

Conservative Party. (2008). *A stronger society: Voluntary action in the 21st century, responsibility agenda* (Policy Green paper No. 5). London: Conservative Party. http://www.conservatives.com/~/media/Files/Green%20Papers/Voluntary_Green_Paper.ashx?dl=true. Accessed 22 February 2010.

Greater London Volunteering. (2010). *Principles of volunteering, originally agreed and endorsed by the London Stakeholders Volunteering Forum and Member of GLV, 2009, Endorsed by the Members of GLV, 2010.* Document available on the webpages of Greater London Volunteering. http://greaterlondonvolunteering.files.wordpress.com/2011/02/principlesofvolunteering.doc. Accessed 12 June 2022.

Grotz, J. (2009). *The dignity and art of voluntary action—Voluntary action, a human value or a commodity.* Paper delivered at ARNOVA's 38th Annual Conference, November 19–22, 2009, Cleveland, Ohio, USA.

Grotz, J. (2010). *When volunteering goes wrong: Misconduct in volunteering.* Paper delivered at 16th NCVO/VSSN Researching the Voluntary Sector Conference, 6–7th September 2010, University of Leeds, UK.

Grotz, J. (2011). *Divisive, harmful and fatal: Less recognised impacts of volunteering.* Paper delivered at the NCVO/VSSN "Researching the Voluntary Sector" Conference 7–8 September 2011, London.

Grotz, J., & Locke, M. (2022). *Volunteers and the law' versus 'volunteer rights,* Paper delivered at Voluntary Action History Society 7th International Conference, 13–15 July 2022, Liverpool.

Grotz, J., Ledgard, M., & Poland, F. (2020). *Patient and public involvement in health and social care: An introduction to theory and practice.* Imprint Springer Nature and Palgrave Macmillan.

Illich, I. (1968). *Untitled talk delivered Saturday April 20 at St. Mary's Lake of the Woods Seminary in Niles (Chicago) Illinois, the talk is also referred to as 'to hell with good intentions'.* A text version of the speech was scanned from an original mimeograph distributed to Conference participants on the following day now available at The Conference on Interamerican Student Projects website. http://www.ciasp.ca/CIASPhistory/IllichCIASPspeech68.pdf. Accessed 26 June 2022.

Institute for Volunteering Research. (1998). *Issues in volunteer management—A report of a survey.* Institute for Volunteering Research.

Johnson, B. (2021). *Prime Minister and head of the NHS call for volunteers to support National Booster Effort*. Press release on the website gov.uk. https://www.gov.uk/government/news/prime-ministeer-and-head-of-the-nhs-call-for-volunteers-to-support-national-booster-effort. Accessed 27 August 2022.

Kruger, D. (2020). *Levelling up our communities: Proposals for a new social covenant A report for government by Danny Kruger MP. A report posted on the website of Danny Kruger MP.* https://www.dannykruger.org.uk/files/2020-09/Kruger%202.0%20Levelling%20Up%20Our%20Communities.pdf. Accessed 26 June 2022.

Lampard, K., & Marsden, E. (2015). *Themes and lessons learnt from NHS investigations into matters relating to Jimmy Savile: Independent report for the Secretary of State for Health.* Report on the website assets.publishing.service.gov.uk. https://assets.publishing.service.gov.uk/government/uploads/system/uploads/attachment_data/file/407209/KL_lessons_learned_report_FINAL.pdf. Accessed 28 May 2020.

Madden, M., & Speed, E. (2017). Beware zombies and unicorns: Toward critical patient and public involvement in health research in a neoliberal context. *Frontiers in Sociology, 2*(7).

McCord, J. (2003). Cures that harm: Unanticipated outcomes of crime prevention programs. *Annals of the American Academy of Political and Social Science, 587*, 16–30.

McGarvey, A., Jochum, V., Chan, O., Delaney, S., Young, R., & Gillies, C. (2020). *Time well spent: Volunteering in the public sector* (Research Report). London: National Council for Voluntary Organisations. https://www.befriending.co.uk/r/24836-time-well-spent-volunteering-in-the-public-sector. Accessed 27 August 2022.

Miliband, E. (2011). *Responsibility in the 21st century*. Transcript of speech on website of politics.co.uk. https://www.politics.co.uk/comment-analysis/2011/06/13/ed-miliband-responsibility-speech-in-full/. Accessed 25 June 2022.

National Council for Voluntary Organisations. (2014). *Final report of the call to action progress group following the volunteer rights inquiry.* National Council for Voluntary Organisations. http://blogs.ncvo.org.uk/wp-content/uploads/mike-locke/call-to-action-progress-group-volunteer-rights-inquiry-report.pdf. Accessed 25 June 2022.

National Council for Voluntary Organisations. (n.d.). *If volunteering goes wrong.* Page on the website of the National Council for Voluntary Organisations. https://www.ncvo.org.uk/get-involved/volunteering/if-volunteering-goes-wrong/. Accessed 27 August 2022.

Putnam, R. D. (2000). *Bowling alone, the collapse and revival of American community*. Simon and Schuster Paperbacks.

Rochester, C., Ellis Paine, A., Howlett, S., with Zimmeck, M. (2010). *Volunteering and society in the 21st century*. Palgrave Macmillan.

Rosenberg, T. (2018). *The business of voluntourism: Do western do-gooders actually do harm?* Contribution on the Guardian website. https://www.theguardian.com/news/2018/sep/13/the-business-of-voluntourism-do-western-do-gooders-actually-do-harm. Accessed 27 August 2022.

Ross, M. W., Greenfield, S. A., & Bennett, L. (1999). Predictors of dropout and burnout in AIDS volunteers: A longitudinal study. *AIDS Care, 11*(6), 723–731.

Smith, D. H. (2000). *Grassroots associations*. Sage.

Smith, D. (2008). Accepting and understanding the dark side of the non profit sector: one key part of building a healthier civil society. Paper delivered at ARNOVA conference November 20–22. Philadelphia, Pennsylvania, USA.

Smith, D. H. (2019). *A review of deviant nonprofit groups: Seeking method in their alleged 'madness-treason-immorality'*. Brill.

Smith, K., & Holmes, K. (2009). Researching volunteers in tourism: Going beyond. *Annals of Leisure Research, 12*(3/4), 403–420.

Stoker, J. (2008). *Report of a review by John Stoker of York Citizens Advice Bureau*. Citizens Advice. http://www.citizensadvice.org.uk/pdf_review_yorkcab_report.pdf. Accessed 31 August 2010.

Teasdale, S. (2008a). *In good health: Assessing the impact of volunteering in the NHS*. Volunteering England.

Teasdale, S. (2008b). *Health check: A practical guide to assessing the impact of volunteering in the NHS*. Volunteering England.

Thoits, P. A., & Hewitt, L. N. (2001). Volunteer work and well-being. *Journal of Health and Social Behavior, 42*(2), 115–131.

Thomas, T. (2022). *Insulate Britain protesters praised by judge who fined them*. News on The Guardian webpages published 13 April 2022. https://www.theguardian.com/environment/2022/apr/13/insulate-britain-protesters-praised-by-judge-who-fined-them. Accessed 28 June 2022.

Tiratelli, L., & Kaye, K. (2020). *Communities vs. coronavirus: The rise of mutual aid*. New Local. https://www.newlocal.org.uk/wp-content/uploads/2020/12/Communities-vs-Coronavirus_New-Local.pdf. Accessed 27 August 2022.

Trades Union Congress. (2009). *A charter for strengthening relations between paid staff and volunteers*. A page on the website of the

Trades Union Congress. https://www.tuc.org.uk/research-analysis/reports/charter-strengthening-relations-between-paid-staff-and-volunteers. Accessed 27 August 2022.

Twigg, J., & Mosel, I. (2017). Emergent groups and spontaneous volunteers in urban disaster response. *Environment and Urbanization, 29*(2), 443–458. https://doi.org/10.1177/0956247817721413. Accessed 28 June 2022.

Unison. (2018a). *Crossing the line, police support volunteers: Rising numbers and mission creep.* Unison. https://www.unison.org.uk/content/uploads/2019/01/Report_on_Police_upport-Volunteers_2018a.pdf. Accessed 12 June 2022.

Unison. (2018b). *Volunteers taking on police roles as cuts continue to bite.* Post on the Unison webpages, 7 December 2018b. https://www.unison.org.uk/news/press-release/2018b/12/volunteers-taking-police-roles-cuts-continue-bite/. Accessed 12 June 2022.

United Nations General Assembly. (2001). *Support for volunteering: Report of the secretary-general.* Page on the website of the United Nations. https://www.un.org/webcast/events/iyv/a56288.pdf. Accessed 27 August 2022.

Volunteer Rights Inquiry. (2010). *Interim report.* Volunteering England. http://www.volunteering.org.uk/NR/rdonlyres/742EBA26-A6CB-4531-BBBB-7C2A35CCE5D5/0/VE_volunteering_inquiry_FIN_web.pdf. Accessed 31 August 2010.

Volunteering England. (2009). *Volunteering England information sheet: If things go wrong.* Volunteering England. http://www.volunteering.org.uk/NR/rdonlyres/BD1C333F-18EF-4FA3-BD66-90780982DF51/0/ISIfThingsGoWrongVE09.pdf. Accessed 31 August 2010.

Volunteering England. (2010). *Volunteer rights inquiry: Interim report.* Volunteering England.

Volunteer Now. (2022). *Working with volunteers—Problem solving procedures.* Page on the website of Volunteer Now. https://www.volunteernow.co.uk/app/uploads/2022/05/Problem-Solving-Procedures-1.pdf. Accessed 27 August 2022.

Ward, L. (2017). *Charities are asking interns to work 252 hours unpaid. That's a scandal.* News on The Guardian webpages published 30 November 2017. https://www.theguardian.com/voluntary-sector-network/2017/nov/30/charities-interns-unpaid-work-scandal-volunteering-experience. Accessed 16 June 2022.

4

Volunteer Involvement in Practice

Abstract This chapter focuses on the relationships built through volunteer involvement, including the different contributions volunteers make, the contexts in which they are involved and the pathways volunteering relationships take. It encourages the reader to use six 'Exercises' to reflect on their own practice in particular on how they describe the contributions volunteers make and on the key steps to ensuring a positive volunteer experience.

Keywords Relationships · Pathways · Impact

Involving volunteers can be difficult and daunting, as anyone trying to find people to join a trustee board or even just to help at the school fete can attest. The more volunteers become involved the more time-consuming and challenging this can become. There is plenty of advice available, but advice alone doesn't get things done. Those involving volunteers learn by experience that volunteer involvement is based on relationships and people achieving together. Depending on the level of involvement the relationships are:

© The Author(s), under exclusive license to Springer Nature
Switzerland AG 2022
J. Grotz and R. Leonard, *Volunteer Involvement*,
https://doi.org/10.1007/978-3-031-19221-0_4

- between those who volunteer and those who involve volunteers,
- between volunteers and people they volunteer to support,
- between those who seek to influence and direct volunteer involvement and the volunteers,
- between those who involve volunteers and the people the volunteering supports
- and, of course, between volunteers themselves.

Volunteer involvement in practice means making these relationships succeed. Achieving positive ongoing relationships requires consistent, mindful responsiveness to differences. People are different, and environments in which volunteering takes place vary greatly. Volunteer involvement requires responding flexibly to the infinite combinations of different volunteers in such circumstances, always remembering to check relationships continue positively, rather than beginning to quietly break down.

We begin this chapter by exploring roles people might play in volunteer involvement. We then discuss volunteer involvement in a range of organisational settings and conclude the chapter by describing wider approaches to the evaluation of volunteer involvement, in particular, the difference volunteer involvement makes.

Before we start, we would like you to consider where you might see volunteer involvement in practice in Exercise 4.1.

Exercise 4.1

Please think of some examples of where volunteer involvement takes place, including those when volunteer involvement is not through registered charities and where the activity may not be commonly described as volunteer involvement.

4.1 Involving and Being Involved: The Roles People Play

Involving volunteers is individual, innovative and ever-changing. Not all volunteers are the same or want to volunteer in the same way. These differences can be characterised in ways that transcend where volunteering takes place and what activity is being carried out. This is in direct contrast to ways of thinking which are solely concerned with filling vacant volunteering opportunities with the most likely or willing candidates. To explain this further, we have adapted a typology, the coherence model (Grotz et al., 2020), which we also use in Chapter Five, to describe the way volunteers might choose to be involved based on their agency, see Table 4.1.

The first group, 'Initiators' are social activists who get things started. They are committed to being the driver of change they want to see, in order to make things better for people. They will do so by getting on and starting something, bringing together a group of others to make it happen, changing the status quo.

The second group, 'Connectors', are well networked within the community and are crucial in turning the 'Initiator's' dreams into reality. They have the contacts, know the key levers to pull and are motivated by the intrinsic desire to make their communities stronger.

Table 4.1 Initiate, connect, collaborate, complement

Initiat(or)	Connect(or)	Collaborate (associate)	Complement(or)
Seeing the need and building the solution	Supporting the development and iteration of the solution	Getting involved to do what is needed with other's support and development	Coming out to support pre-arranged roles, usually at agreed times and in specific ways
Challenging and transforming	Connecting with others to create infrastructure	Self-directing but within framework of tasks	Enabled by clear structure and boundaries

'Associates', the third group, probably most closely describe the 9% of people carrying out half of the volunteering activities described by Mohan and Bulloch (2012) as the 'civic core'. They step up to do what is needed because they believe it to be right and they are solution finders. They want to do something and need to know it is useful, adding value, interacting when they get a sense of direction of travel they can get behind.

'Complementors' are the fourth group, who want to provide support to others but not be part of the organising or developing aspects. They want to be able to turn up and do what is needed but not be expected to offer more than that, preferring to receive clear guidance or boundaries around their actions. Everything has been sorted out for them already and they just turn up.

Of course, these are coarse categories and they will constantly overlap. Time and circumstances can affect where people fall within these groups. People might have different roles at the same time in different organisations or their roles within a setting might change over time.

Before we go on to consider some implications of conceiving volunteer involvement in this way, we suggest you reflect on the questions in Exercise 4.2 about what roles you have seen or experienced in volunteer involvement.

Exercise 4.2

Reflecting on the four types we have described, where would you put yourself currently? Or in the past? Have you been or are you in more than one of them, and what does that mean for each role?

What would your expectations be of how you'd like to be involved, if you were to consider volunteering?

Whatever people's roles end up being, involving volunteers is based on personal relationships and is best when directly aligned to what individuals want to do and get out of it. This then enables the deeper connections people feel with what they are doing, responding to the complexity of its impact on their lives. This means thinking of developing relationships with people where they are, valuing and incorporating their strengths and assets with an existing community, empowering people to use these to shape solutions within supportive relationships.

In some instances, particularly within contexts which are entirely volunteer-led and delivered, it can mean that volunteers take on more than they had originally expected or signed up for, such as, not only being responsible for involving volunteers themselves and the logistics around that, but also the finance, training, complaint handling and, in some cases, property and even staff management. 'Connectors' might relish this and will be keen to develop through this experience, while others might feel more of a sense of duty: 'if they don't who will?'. The opportunity to organise can be offered to those who have skills and expressed an interest, irrespective of whether or how they are involved with the core offer.

Another aspect of involving volunteers that sometimes occurs is the tension between volunteers being able to specialise and focus on tasks but at the same time wanting to do more or different things being able to innovate and experiment. Over one in six volunteers said they have skills and experience which they'd like to use in volunteering but are not currently using (McGarvey et al., 2019, p. 50).

Recognising the different types of volunteer involvement is essential for giving a positive and effective volunteer involvement experience. From having a vision and starting a social movement, as 'Initiators', to carrying out ongoing day-to-day tasks as 'Complementors', and those who involve volunteers needing to align these roles appropriately to someone's individual motivations, volunteer involvement can take place without the conscious direction of a constituted organisation, and often does. Many of the current registered organisations grew out of a community movement based on the idea of someone volunteering in the style of 'Initiators' who with the assistance of 'Connectors' created links and structures to keep it sustainable, maintained and developed by 'Associate' volunteers, with 'on the ground' activities being carried out by those who we categorised as 'Complementors'.

4.2   Agency Within Agencies

As people volunteer for different causes in types of environments, we will explore how this might be supported within seven different environments.

4.2.1 VCSE with no Paid Staff

Volunteering involvement is often associated with activities in the Voluntary, Community and Social Enterprise sector, such as in a registered charity. This is sometimes referred to as the Third sector, civil society or the not-for-profit sector. At the time of writing, August 2022, the Charity Commission records that there are over 183,954 charities in England and Wales, with 925,254 trustees and 5,259,280 volunteers (Charity Commission, 2022). Charities' activities are directed by their objects as set out in their statutes, and they are governed by a board of trustees, who are also volunteers. They act as autonomous bodies but need to abide by legislative processes. The majority of these organisations have no paid staff and volunteers tend to be involved in all the elements of governance and day-to-day delivery of activities. There might be dedicated tasks, like taking the lead on finding and supporting new volunteers or for keeping in touch with volunteers.

4.2.2 VCSE with Paid Staff

In August 2022, the Charity Commission (2022) reports 1,060,269 employees of charities, an apparent increase from the paid workforce of 951,611 previously reported in the Civil Society Almanac of the National Council for Voluntary Organisations (2021). In many cases, staff in these organisations direct volunteering activities and organise the involvement of volunteers. In some cases, paid staff are specifically employed to enable and ensure continuous and consistent volunteer involvement. There could be an entire team which sets strategic direction and ensures a consistent experience for all volunteers within the organisation. Such a team is likely to take into consideration legal and safeguarding obligations, including police checks of potential volunteers where necessary or ensuring appropriate money handling processes. In other cases, involving volunteers can be a part of a staff member's broader role, which might also include fundraising duties and running operations. Many of the volunteering activities which take place in VCSE organisations with paid staff are prescribed and, while there may be flexibility in how they are carried out, they are likely to fall within a programme of activities directed by a staff team as opposed to being developed and led by volunteers themselves. Most of the volunteers within these organisations are likely to be those who fall into the 'Complementors' category so are happy to turn up and carry out their task. In some cases, they are led by volunteers with 'Associate' characteristics who want to take more of an organising role, seeking a stronger involvement with the cause. Trustees are volunteers, so those who take on this role within organisations which have paid staff are likely to be Connectors, as are any other function or group which is involved in shaping the operational direction.

4.2.3 VCSE with Staff and Volunteer-Led Branches, Groups

About a third of UK-wide charities are formed from a network of local branches. Many of these branches are run autonomously by volunteers linked to a staff team which cascades advice and guidance to their local network. In some organisations, these branches are independent legal entities brought together in a national or regional federated structure. Staff members in the structure may set a central process and procedures for branches to follow, and offer training on all aspects of managing a branch including volunteer involvement. The volunteers who lead the local branches are likely to be 'Connectors' using their organisational skills and relationships to run the group, turning centralised guidance into day-to-day practice. They are likely to involve a core group of people who are often 'Associates' to support the activities and ensure logistics happen through 'Complementors' who turn up to carry out tasks, as required. There is likely to be the opportunity for 'Initiators' to be able to influence and create new ways of involving, through the nationally federated structure of volunteer-led branches.

4.2.4   Public Services

Increasingly statutory organisations are recognising the value of involving volunteers, such as in health and social care or criminal justice, with many having well-established volunteering schemes, supported by specific staff roles. Local Authorities also have long-held relationships, including official partnerships, with the voluntary, community and more recently social enterprise sectors to help provide care services. For those who volunteer within statutory agencies, there appears to be reduced opportunity to be anything other than directed with tasks being allocated to them, so they are more likely to be attractive to 'Complementors' and 'Associates'. But even they may feel that their volunteering is overly bureaucratic (McGarvey et al., 2020, p. 31).

There are emerging cases of local authorities who now recognise the benefit of collaborating in a more flexible way with local communities and self-organising groups such as those involved with 'New Local' an independent think tank and network of local councils with "*a mission to transform public services and unlock community power*", chaired by Donna Hall (New Local, 2022). This particular network aims to enable people to contribute their existing strengths to solving local problems including transferring assets to communities. Volunteer involvement is increasingly seen as a powerful way of supporting this.

4.2.5   Private Business

One way for the private or for-profit sector to demonstrate their desire to implement corporate social responsibility as well as to provide positive development opportunities for their staff is through employer supported volunteering (ESV). This may be carried out via a national charity or local community group and can sometimes be provided in the form of a financial contribution, such as within a corporate partnership. Results from a national survey in 2015 showed that about 5% of employees volunteered in this way (Chartered Institute of Personnel & Development, 2015, p. 3).

Traditionally, these relationships were conceived as team building 'paint and fix' exercises, such as a local firm painting a community centre, but more recently they have been morphing into skill sharing opportunities such as a company's finance team advising a local charity on financial strategy. There could also be opportunities for employees to volunteer with delivery or operational activities. Charities are also collaborating more closely with the private sector to develop bespoke options that serve both parties better. ESV seems best when the purpose of the volunteer involving organisation and the employer align. It becomes better if they build good relationships at different levels, have a shared understanding of aims, and agree on where and how to handover responsibility for volunteer involvement.

Community businesses also involve volunteers and some of them depend on volunteers, including enterprises which are closely linked to providing public services such as community libraries. Recent research identified three main reasons for involving volunteers in community businesses: resource, reflection of ethos and value, and also as a way to build legitimacy and distinction (Ellis Paine et al., 2021, p. 23).

4.2.6 Volunteering Infrastructure Organisations

Volunteering infrastructure organisations such as Councils for Voluntary Service and Volunteer Centres within England and Third Sector Interfaces within Scotland provide support and advice on all aspects of volunteer involvement and other organisational development as well as support around running groups such as capacity building, building systems or generating income. They help with promoting volunteering opportunities and matching people with these, offering training on involving volunteers and also to volunteers, providing guidance and templates for key policies. They bring together groups, representing them and advocating on their behalf at local or regional levels, as well as amplifying the voice of volunteers in discussions with other stakeholders such as local authorities, for example, when considering local volunteering strategies (Grotz et al., 2022). Often involving others, these are a good place for 'Connectors' to create links and 'Initiators' to shape ideas. 'Associates' and 'Complementors' will be able to find out more about where they can get involved in more practical, direct delivery ways.

4.2.7 Associations

It is likely that most volunteer involvement happens outside an established organisational structure with people using their own initiative, addressing the issues or meeting needs within their own communities. Mutual Aid expressly *"aims to transgress the hierarchies of established charities and erase distinctions between helpers and helped in order to prefigure a more equal—and stateless—society"* (Preston & Firth, 2020, p. 57). This communitarian activity has always been there but became more publicly recognised during the COVID-19 pandemic with the seeming proliferation of mutual aid groups.

> Mutual aid is where a group of people organise to meet their own needs, outside of the formal frameworks of charities, NGOs and government. It is, by definition, a horizontal mode of organising, in which all individuals are equally powerful. There are no 'leaders' or unelected 'steering committees' in mutual aid projects; there is only a group of people who work together as equals. (Covid-19 Mutual Aid, 2020)

Despite the perceived lack of structure of associations, such as community and mutual aid groups, there is still likely to be an organising principle, with responsibilities shared in the involvement of volunteers (Power & Benton, 2021), which has its own particular challenges. Their supporting framework can be developed as helpful guidance rather than aiming to regulate the element of self-organising into something more bureaucratic.

People with a high desire for autonomy and independence will identify need and start up such groups, so tend to be 'Initiators'. This is the case whether the action is mobilising others in the face of an emergency or taking over a library threatened with closure. Unless this act is solely being carried out alone, 'Initiators' will go on to involve others and 'Connectors' will be best placed to bring people and resources together. If anything further is needed, 'Associates' can organise and 'Complementors' will come on board to carry out any tasks.

Regardless of the type of group or organisation in which volunteer involvement takes place there are key elements to consider. According to the 2019 'Time Well Spent' Research by NCVO, over a third (35%) of the volunteer respondents think their volunteering could be better organised. Yet, around one quarter (24%) think that there is too much bureaucracy (McGarvey et al., 2019). This point provides those who want to involve volunteers with something to consider, especially as, the research points out, this is something which was also noted in the 'Helping Out Survey' undertaken 15 years previously (Low et al., 2007). How do we ensure the necessary and relevant structures without impeding the volunteer experience? This is particularly relevant as another concern from nearly a fifth (19%) of the respondents in the NCVO research is that volunteering is becoming too much like 'paid work'. The overarching element of volunteer involvement is relationship building and ensuring there's a chance to offer a person-centred meaningful opportunity, which may change or evolve throughout the volunteer's involvement with the organisation or sector.

Before we next look specifically at relationship building, we suggest you to consider the question in Exercise 4.3 on how you might prepare for involving volunteers.

Exercise 4.3

What is most important when you are thinking about involving volunteers?

4.3 Relationship Pathways

Bringing together the structure which supports and enables volunteer involvement within such diverse locations and contexts, with the individuality of people using their own assets within their own lives and communities, is challenging. Any structure needs to be flexible enough to not get in the way of the self-organising and volunteer-led aspect, to "*not crush the butterfly within the jam jar*", as the 'Relationship Project' puts it (Robinson, 2020, p. 19), such as not to lose the wonder and intrinsic value of volunteering by trying to over-regulate it.

The resources that can be put into volunteer involvement will be dependent on what the organisation has available but there are key elements to be aware of. This is mainly around creating and maintaining good relationships. One of the findings from 'Pathways through Participation' was that while volunteering is an essential element of participation, it was not easy to actually become involved.

> People often lack information and knowledge about opportunities to participate and support mechanisms available at the local level (....) Far more needs to be done to publicise volunteer opportunities especially to wider audiences and through a variety of means. (Brodie et al., 2011, p. 2)

A volunteering opportunity will need to be clearly described and actively discussed, so that people who want to become involved know what is needed and how they will be part of the process. Word of mouth and just asking people to come along is an excellent way for volunteers and those wanting to involve them to find each other. It is seen as possibly the most effective way to begin volunteer involvement (Low et al., 2007; Brodie et al., 2011, p. 70). But by using word of mouth, those who want to involve volunteers will need to take extra care that they do not inadvertently exclude people by only involving 'people like me'. Relationships are best built by being where people are. If volunteers can see that what they're already doing is seen as valuable, and understand what further opportunities there are, it will be easier to collaborate to explore how further involvement can fit into their lives and interests.

Being able to have a shared agreement and understanding of how volunteers will be involved helps to develop a positive and effective relationship, and is best gained early on. Reflecting on the different expectations which individuals will have regarding limits to what needs doing, thoughts on how to best meet needs, and volunteers' varying desire for agency means that the perspectives of each side need to be explored and understood. Research looking at psychological contract theory as a way to better understand how to involve volunteers identified concerns regarding differing expectations from volunteers as well as from the organisations that sought to involve them (Ralston et al 2004). If expectations are aligned, both volunteers and those involving them may decide to continue the relationship (Delaney, 2014, p. 9).

This means ensuring good opportunities for both parties to discuss what the volunteer wants to get out of being involved. Conversations can establish how volunteers or the organisation prefer the activities to be carried out, as well as an overview of what is likely to be expected, and what the opportunity to shape activities undertaken will be. This will empower volunteers to make more informed decisions and also potentially help the volunteer involving organisation to be better informed when planning future possible activities, as such ideas can be shared.

Much of this relates to volunteer motivations so before moving on, we suggest you to consider the question in Exercise 4.4 about when you would start taking into account volunteer motivation.

Exercise 4.4

When does thinking about volunteer motivation start? Is it:

- when volunteers are leaving,
- as you first meet them,
- or before you start sending out information for a volunteer activity?

Motivations can be one of the topics which are easily overlooked but understanding them will help to plan more effectively for the involvement of volunteers. Not just when considering the wider appeal to encourage people to get in touch initially, but also reflecting during all stages of the involvement process, which means being able to build in a personalised relationship with volunteers, linking with individual preferences.

'Initiators' will want to have full autonomy over what they do. They are likely to take the lead in developing and creating new initiatives and will want to be enabled to do this easily.

'Connectors' are those who will support and develop the structures and build the key relationships needed to keep the project or service running. They want to be part of shaping the route so will be motivated by being offered opportunities to do this, taking on important leadership positions within the setting, group or organisation.

'Associates' are motivated by taking responsibility for their actions within a parameter that has been pre-set. These are often the volunteers that are relied on to get things done and while this might be a factor which they value, it is important not to take these particular volunteers for granted. Regular check-ins are important to avoid disappointment. Associates can play a role within all volunteer involving models.

'Complementors' want to know that they are able to turn up and do what is required and that this action has made a difference. They do not want to feel that their time has been wasted and may feel frustrated if things are not organised well, so knowing and understanding their expectations is important.

Of course it is worth emphasising that these are generalisations and as the research for 'Pathways through Participation' showed, involvement processes are dynamic.

> ...people's involvement changes over their life course as they experience different life events and triggers; there are periods of time when barriers are more prevalent and others when enabling factors have a greater role to play. (Brodie et al., 2011, p. 6)

Building a relationship with volunteers means it will be possible to recognise how these needs change and it's also a way to keep people informed with any relevant news. Before we move on, we suggest you have a look at the questions in Exercise 4.5 and consider how you could make sure volunteers are staying up-to-date.

> **Exercise 4.5**
>
> How do you ensure your volunteers know what's going on; what's happening both at a local level and throughout any wider organisation? How are volunteers able to feed their views into any development?

Whatever role someone carries out, they are likely to want to know what's going on, and ultimately what difference they've made. It is worth considering how to communicate this to volunteers. How do they prefer to be kept up-to-date and what methods are best for them? Good communication is at the root of volunteer involvement and gives people a "sense of belonging" (Jackson et al., 2019, p. 201).

Communication needs to be two-way. Some volunteers will want to be able to interact with and feed into any group setting. 'Initiators' and 'Connectors' will want to do this more actively, particularly with regard to how they can add value, and others will prefer a more structured mechanism.

The voice of volunteers brings credibility to an organisation or cause, and while 'Initiators' and 'Connectors' will be motivated by being part of these conversations, the voices of 'Associates' and 'Complementors' can also be brought in through a more structured manner to ensure that their voices are integrated into any process.

Any setup for communication should have a space for discussion. It is reasonable and sometimes necessary to ask that public comments made on behalf of an organisation or group are aligned with its strategy and direction but as part of that, there should be an opportunity for volunteers and other stakeholders to feed into the internal conversation.

Volunteers will want to know, at a minimum, that what they have done has benefitted the cause they have been supporting and they might also expect something in return, such as feelings of "*friendship, satisfaction, influence, support, confidence, skills and recognition*" (Brodie et al., 2011, p. 37).

Being able to show the value of someone's involvement is part of keeping a relationship. So before moving on, have a look at Exercise 4.6 and consider how you might show a volunteer you value them.

Exercise 4.6

What ideas do you have about how to show you value volunteers?

People generally don't seem to expressly ask to be thanked or shown appreciation but if this 'hygiene factor' is lacking, then that will be noticed. Nobody wants to feel unappreciated or, even worse, taken advantage of. Thanking someone in simple ways such as sending a personal email following an activity, including an update on what this has achieved through their efforts, can be powerful.

Developing a better understanding of what an individual volunteer wants to get out of their involvement and making sure there are appropriate ongoing efforts made to demonstrate that they are valued, as well as exploring how they can be more, less or differently involved matters hugely. It could be that someone who has been carrying out a predetermined activity would like to be more involved in supporting others and leading. Just being able to offer that option to them is a sign that they are recognised. Of course, it could be the opposite. A volunteer who used to thrive at key leadership roles might like to step back and finding a way of seeing and enabling this to happen will help to show that they are valued for who they are, not just for what they do for the group. Feeling undervalued can be a source of concern and complaint for volunteers but actions can be taken and planned, to mitigate against such negative aspects of volunteer involvement.

When collaborating with any group of people, it is simply inevitable that something will go wrong, not only as differences of expectation or disparate points of view emerge. Even with community volunteer-led groups, there may be issues, as the New Local Government Network found in their research on mutual aid groups. They learnt that despite successes during the COVID-19 pandemic, many newly established groups *"have encountered a range of challenges, from managing the conduct and morale of volunteers"* (Tiratelli & Kaye, 2020, p. 21). This is also bearing out evidence from 'Pathways through Participation' that *"insular or cliquey groups and organisations had caused some (of their interviewees) to stop their participation"* (Brodie et al., 2011, p. 44).

Some observers suggest that the power of volunteering comes to the fore when it is free to explore alternative answers to problems and not just seen as an option which fits into a pre-determined solution. Matthew Syed writes in his 2019 book 'Rebel Ideas' *"wise groups…bring insights from different regions of the problem space. Such groups contain people with perspectives that challenge, augment, diverge and cross-pollinate"* (Syed, 2019, p. 54). The diversity of thought offered by a group of people who are not inculcated into a system is valuable and the courage which is needed to support this is an element that needs to be embedded, meaningfully, within any framework which wants to encourage volunteering. However, this remains a challenge, as a report on 'Diversity and Volunteering' illustrates, with some groups of volunteers not having positive volunteering experiences because of barriers relating to organisational culture, attitudes and lack of flexibility (Donahue et al., 2020, p. 38).

Flexibility, simplicity of access and being more proactive in how volunteers are brought together as unique individuals to create an inclusive culture will benefit all. 'Connectors' will value being part of developing this. 'Complementors' and 'Associates' will approve the fact that that their time isn't being wasted but the latter will need to have clear guidelines so that the process doesn't feel too aimless.

It is also important to give people permission to stop volunteering! It is much more motivating to know that you can leave if you want to and that you can do so positively. A culture that solely reflects length and amount of time involved is not necessarily attractive. Having an open and appreciative response, enabling people to move away will be more likely to mean a volunteer will return if circumstances change, and also for them to recommend volunteering to families or friends.

4.4   Measuring Impact: Knowing the Difference You Make

It might be a bit surprising, but even in the business magazine 'Forbes', Field (2016) suggests that 'measuring impact is good for business'.

> For social entrepreneurs, impact investors, of course, are a crucial source of funding. So, probably goes without saying that whatever can create the most value for such investors likely is also a good thing for mission-driven ventures.

The difference made by an activity like volunteering is often referred to as 'impact'. Impact is not seen as the financial bottom line but relates to the changes an activity engenders over time. As Field above suggests, being able to show evidence of impact has become an important component in volunteer involvement, especially when justifying funding or seeking investment. Other rationales to undertake an evaluation include improving services, strategic planning or assessing whether targets set by a public sector funder have been achieved.

Determining what is worth evaluating can be vexing and a serious criticism can be that the impact of volunteer involvement is not necessarily vigorously assessed, with programmes looking simply for positive results. At the very core of assessing impact, we should be seeking to objectively understand the differences an activity makes, good, bad or none at all, and this requires a systematic approach. As with 'volunteer involvement', people don't necessarily agree on how to undertake an evaluation or what to call its components. We cannot discuss evaluations in detail but will look at outcomes to illustrate the basic idea.

4.4.1 Towards Outcomes

There are different techniques to evaluating impact. They each have value in different circumstances. We will briefly introduce just one of them, the use of a logic model in evaluation, which requires planning. Possibly the most important thing to remember, you cannot effectively impose a logic model on something that has not been logically planned and it is therefore almost impossible to impose it retrospectively, once what is going to be evaluated has already happened. It means you have to start by thinking about evaluations or at least include it in you early planning.

In the 1970s, evaluators like Carol Weiss (1972) began developing logic models which have since become used in specific techniques such as in developing a 'Theory of Change'. To create a logic model, you first collaboratively establish what your problem is and what success would look like if the problem is resolved. For example, if there is no natural and leisure environment in your area and you want to help to create one, do you therefore want to restore a forest or a canal, improving the environment? Or are you looking at an area of deprivation and your overarching aim is for the volunteers you involve to benefit by improved well-being or employability? The steps you need to take to achieve your aim will differ depending on the aim. Next, you need to clearly identify the different steps you have to take to make the changes you want to achieve, and only then, can you start to design the actions that will affect the changes, which in turn you hope will address your problem. This means the beginning of your evaluation coincides with your action planning, and it guides the way you will measure them later, once delivered. In a logic model, the results of your actions are often referred to as 'outputs', the changes you achieve are referred to as 'outcomes', and if after all that you can identify long-term changes that happen, helping to address the overall problem, you might have impact, see Fig. 4.1.

Once you have clarified the steps that may lead to your intended impact, you can consider what can be measured and how, within such a

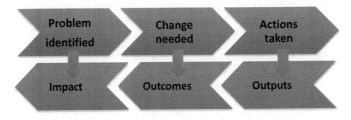

Fig. 4.1 'Basic logic model', is based on Grotz et al. (2020)

model. It is usually helpful to cut the big problem into many little pieces and see how addressing them will contribute to solving the big problem. People use different matrices but they are likely to connect the following parts:

Aims	What needs to be achieved overall to resolve your problem?
Objectives	What are the specific areas to be addressed and the actions you will take?
Indicators	What does success look like when you achieve those aims?
Measures	How to know whether the aims were achieved?

4.4.2 Assessing What Counts, Attaching Values

However, using a logic model and a matrix to determine measures, or similar techniques are only tools to help assess the difference any planned activity makes. They are not a means to attach particular value and they may not capture all differences made, especially if the overall aim is an elusive concept. Geoff Mulgan at 'Nesta', for example, acknowledges challenges when assessing the impact of innovation.

> The measurement of innovation impact is rarely straightforward but it's essential to try and track what is being achieved" …"persuading a small group of decision makers to change their mind can sometimes be far more impactful than an opinion piece in a newspaper read by millions. (Mulgan, no date)

This means the clearer and realistic your overall aim, the more chance you have to connect the dots logically. When evaluating impact and attaching values, we can also distinguish between what values are and who they might be for. Values might be 'physical' such as an enhanced environment, 'cultural' such as events and sense of belonging, 'social' such as stronger associations involving more people, 'human' such as new skills or more confidence or 'economic' including increased income. Using the 'Volunteering Impact Assessment Toolkit' developed by the Institute for Volunteering Research, first published in 2004, Thomas (2006) assessed the impact of volunteering in a London borough as perceived by the volunteers themselves, on themselves and on the beneficiaries. There are also ways of attributing economic value to volunteering, such as with a calculator to assess benefits of employer supported volunteering (Connolly & Woodard, 2022).

4.5 Summary and Conclusion

Volunteers are different. They differ in their needs and expectations, in the places in which they volunteer and in the ways they become involved. We need to ensure that the environment to support volunteer involvement can respond appropriately to such differences. There is 'no one size fits all' approach to the practice of volunteer involvement. In this, and within all environments in which volunteering takes place, developing personalised relationships to better understand what people need is vital. But even within complex situations, volunteer involvement can be light touch, offering quick and easy entry routes with flexibility to allow agency and self-efficacy, explaining, discussing and agreeing clear expectations of everyone involved, and explaining the opportunity for enjoyment, mutual benefit and reciprocity.

Good communication and building on an understanding of people's individual needs and motivations are key ingredients, underpinning appropriate levels of support and information and are part of the ongoing relationship when involving volunteers. This creates a balance between an efficient, safe and supportive process and a personal, responsive and adaptable relationship.

References

Brodie, E., Hughes, T., Jochum, V., Miller, S., Ockenden, N., & Warburton, D. (2011). *Pathways through participation: What creates and sustains active citizenship?* NCVO, IVR, involve. https://involve.org.uk/resources/public ations/project-reports/pathways-through-participation. Accessed 27 August 2022.

Chartered Institute of Personnel and Development. (2015). *On the brink of a game-changer? Building sustainable partnerships between companies and voluntary organisations*. Chartered Institute of Personnel and Development, IVR. https://www.cipd.co.uk/Images/on-brink-game-changer_2015_tcm18-9047.pdf. Accessed 27 August 2022.

Charity Commission. (2022). *Charities in England and Wales—27 August 2022*. Information on the website of the Charity Commission. https://register-of-charities.charitycommission.gov.uk/sector-data/sector-overview. Accessed 27 August 2022.

Connolly, S., & Woodard, R. (2022). *The value of values: Calculating the economic and individual benefits of workplace volunteering*. Blog on the website of the Institute for Volunteering Research. https://www.uea.ac.uk/web/groups-and-centres/institute-for-volunteering-research/blog. Accessed 27 August 2022.

Covid-19 Mutual Aid UK. (2020). *Frequently asked questions*. Page on the website of COVID-19 Mutual Aid UK. https://covidmutualaid.org/faq/. Accessed 27 June 2022.

Delaney, S. (2014). *Making a big deal out of it, understanding volunteer management through applying psychological contract theory*. Paper on website of Voluntary Sector Studies Network, from VSSN Conference 2014 New researchers' sessions. http://www.vssn.org.uk/wp-content/uploads/2014/10/Abstract-and-paper-Shaun-Delaney.pdf. Accessed 28 August 2022.

Donahue, K., McGarvey, A., Rooney, K., & Jochum, V. (2020). *Time well Spent: Diversity and volunteering research report December 2020*. National Council for Voluntary Organisations. https://ncvo-app-wagtail-mediaa721a567-uwkfinin077j.s3.amazonaws.com/documents/time_well_spent_diversity_and_volunteering_final.pdf. Accessed 28 August 2022]

Ellis Paine, A., Damm, C., Dean, J., Harris, C., & Macmillan, R. (2021). *Volunteering in community business: Meaning, practice and management*. Centre for Regional Economic and Social Research. https://www.shu.ac.uk/-/media/home/research/cresr/reports/v/volunteering-in-community-business.pdf. Accessed 27 June 2022.

Field, A. (2016). *Why measuring impact is good for business*. Contribution on Forbes Magazine website. https://www.forbes.com/sites/annefield/2016/08/28/why-measuring-impact-is-good-for-business/?sh=10e8c67d7ddf. Accessed 27 August 2022.

Grotz, J., Ledgard, M., & Poland, F. (2020). *Patient and public involvement in health and social care: An introduction to theory and practice*. Imprint Springer Nature and Palgrave Macmillan.

Grotz, J., Connolly, S., Woodard, R., & Parkinson, E. (2022). *Volunteering voices: A future vision for Hastings*. Institute for Volunteering Research.

Jackson, R., Locke, M., Hogg, E., & Lynch, R. (2019). *The complete volunteer management handbook* (4th ed.). Directory of Social Change.

Low, N., Butt, S., Ellis Paine, A., & Davis-Smith, J. (2007). *Helping out: A national survey of volunteering and charitable giving*. Cabinet Office.

McGarvey, A., Jochum, V., Chan, O., Delaney, S., Young, R., & Gillies, C. (2020). *Time well spent: Volunteering in the public sector* (Research Report). London: National Council for Voluntary Organisations. https://www.befriending.co.uk/r/24836-time-well-spent-volunteering-in-the-public-sector. Accessed 27 August 2022.

McGarvey, A., Jochum, V., Davies, J., Dobbs, J., & Hornung, L. (2019). *Time well spent: A national survey on the volunteer experience*. NCVO.

Mohan, J., & Bulloch, S. L. (2012). *The idea of a 'civic core': What are the overlaps between charitable giving, volunteering, and civic participation in England and Wales?* (Third Sector Research Centre Working Paper 73). https://www.birmingham.ac.uk/Documents/college-social-sciences/social-policy/tsrc/working-papers/working-paper-73.pdf. Accessed 27 August 2022.

National Council for Voluntary Organisations. (2021). *UK Civil Society Almanac 2021: Data trends insights*. Executive summary on webpages of National Council for Voluntary Organisations. https://www.ncvo.org.uk/news-and-insights/news-index/uk-civil-society-almanac-2021/. Accessed 27 August 2022.

New Local. (2022). *About*. Page in the website of New Local. www.newlocal.org.uk/about/. Accessed 29 August 2022.

Power, A., & Benton, E. (2021). *Where next for Britain's 4,300 mutual aid groups?* Blog on the website of LSE. https://blogs.lse.ac.uk/covid19/2021/05/06/where-next-for-britains-4300-mutual-aid-groups/. Accessed 27 August 2022.

Preston, J., & Firth, R. (2020). *Coronavirus, class and mutual aid in the United Kingdom*. Palgrave Macmillan.

Ralston, D., Downward, P. & Lundsdon, L. (2004). The expectations of volunteers prior to the XVII Commonwealth Games, 2002: A qualitative study, *Event Management*, 9(1–2), pp. 1–2.

Robinson, D. (2020). *The moment we noticed: The relationships observatory and our learning from 100 days of lockdown*. Relationships Project. https://relationshipsproject.org/content/uploads/2020/07/The-Moment-We-Noticed_RelationshipsProject_202.pdf. Accessed 27 August 2022.

Syed, M. (2019). *Rebel ideas: The power of diverse thinking*. John Murray.

Thomas, B. (2006). Assessing the impact of volunteering in a London borough. *Voluntary Action, 8*(1), 92–103.

Tiratelli, L., & Kaye, K. (2020). *Communities vs. coronavirus: The rise of mutual aid*. New Local. https://www.newlocal.org.uk/wp-content/uploads/2020/12/Communities-vs-Coronavirus_New-Local.pdf. Accessed 27 August 2022.

Weiss, C. H. (1972). *Evaluation research: Methods for assessing program effectiveness*. Prentice Hall.

5

Reflective Volunteer Involvement

Abstract Chapter Five introduces the concept of reflective volunteer involvement, discussing how volunteers and those who seek to involve them can find and understand each other, how they agree ways to act together and how they can know that they are making a difference. It offers nine 'Practice Examples' illustrating the important role of communicating, supporting and valuing.

Keywords Reflective · Connecting · Collaborating

Volunteer involvement is complex and ever-changing. In order to succeed, it needs action which is reflective. It is not an industrial process where action A automatically and in standard ways leads to outcome B. Making relationships succeed requires recognising levels of autonomy, agreeing actions and making a difference together. In this chapter, we seek to combine what we have set out regarding theory and practice so far, suggesting some key steps that might be helpful when involving volunteers. To place order on the many components, we apply the 'coherence model' of public and partner involvement (Grotz et al., 2020).

© The Author(s), under exclusive license to Springer Nature
Switzerland AG 2022
J. Grotz and R. Leonard, *Volunteer Involvement*,
https://doi.org/10.1007/978-3-031-19221-0_5

This includes attending to and developing ways of connecting, collaborating and complementing. Connecting is the process of volunteers and those who seek to involve them finding and understanding each other, collaborating requires agreeing ways to act together and complementing is making a difference together. We will provide nine brief case studies to illustrate some challenges in volunteer involvement, which relate to reflectively communicating, valuing and monitoring. However, this is not a rule book. We offer some practical steps within this chapter as starting points for anyone who is involving volunteers, to reflect on how their actions and resources for connecting, collaborating and complementing may more effectively ensure a good experience for everyone.

5.1   Connecting

In this section, we will explore how to start the volunteer involvement, by building well-founded relationships to make sure that everyone involved is ready and confident to begin volunteering. To better understand why and how people come together, we need to reflect on the motivations and needs of everyone involved and carefully consider our actions. We will be looking in particular at:

* Planning volunteer involvement,
* Finding opportunities and volunteers,
* Understanding each other.

5.1.1 Planning Volunteer Involvement

Reflecting on volunteer involvement before it begins, thinking through the first steps, is as important as to plan for the long term, to ensure such involvement is initially acceptable and sustainable. Also, if involvement has not been logically planned and thought through, a logic model as a basis for evaluating an activity is unlikely to achieve its purpose.

Planning, including volunteer involvement, does not have to mean one or a few people directing activities in a top-down approach. Involving volunteers in a way which fits the spirit of inclusive volunteering is predicated on building good personal relationships. Even informal groups or activities must still generate an atmosphere welcoming to all and this doesn't just happen, but takes dedicated resources and consideration. To ensure positive and meaningful volunteering experiences requires forethought, enabling everyone who involves volunteers to feel comfortable and confident in their abilities and to be or become sufficiently knowledgeable about how to engage with an individual's and community's assets. This includes taking the time to make sure that the key elements for successful involvement are either present or there are plans to develop them.

A volunteer journey must be keeping a balance between efficiently providing support for volunteers, commensurate with the activities and ensuring relationships between people and organisations, remaining adaptable and responsive all the way through. Once involved, volunteers need to be supported, in a way that is meaningful to them and meets their changing needs. Groups or organisations which involve volunteers may also have priorities which change, and that needs to be shared or better still co-produced with everyone involved. Resources need to be available to support volunteer involvement, including ensuring that responsibilities are defined for leading, enabling or supporting volunteer involvement on an ongoing basis.

The group or organisation will have a range of needs which will vary across the diverse volunteer involving activities, from the autonomous volunteer community activist to the volunteer in a specialist programme in a national charity. Offering activities which meet these needs in similarly diverse ways will extend an organisation's reach and increase everyone's creativity.

Volunteer involving organisations, large or small, with paid staff or completely volunteer-led often say that they want more volunteers. However, before just starting to bring people in, it is important to know how to meaningfully involve them and understand what would motivate someone to become involved with the offer. We've reflected that people have different needs, and that these may change throughout their lives, so ensure these can fit in by offering a variety of opportunities.

Hearing from volunteers directly and keeping them involved and updated individually in any development is important. Can resource be put towards ensuring no one will be out-of-pocket as well as for thanking and celebrating their involvement? And supporting someone to stop volunteering if that's right for them, without impacting anyone who might be receiving support from them will need consideration.

Any planning should include contingencies to assess risks and ensure safeguarding. What steps can be put in place to try to prevent any problems or make things right if things do go wrong? Capturing such things in writing so they can be shared and agreed to is useful and there are templates for policies and processes available online and a local Centre for Voluntary Service will be able to offer help with planning. Only once you've carefully considered how you will support volunteer involvement might you be ready to start finding volunteers.

Practice Example: One

'A' lived by the coast and was keen on ensuring that the family did something to support the environment. He saw a poster promoting a beach clean and looked online for more details. Registering to attend was quick and easy and the system allowed him to choose whether his details could be saved for future or nearby activities. The details given were clear about where to turn up and how long the activity was likely to be. When 'A' signed up, he was sent information about who to contact on the day and told that litter pickers and bags would be available. Initially concerned that he'd be asked to do more than he was willing to, 'A' was reassured that the organisation would only contact him to tell him the results of the day's activities. Pleased at the simplicity of getting involved and how it had been a positive way to make a difference with his sons 'A' willingly signed up for the next litter pick and offered to extend his involvement to carry out the survey of what was collected as well.

5.1.2 Finding Opportunities and Volunteers

Finding volunteers is often flagged up by those who involve volunteers, as one of the issues that concerns them most. We know this from our personal experience as trustee board chairs. Yet, there are many people looking for places and ways to get involved, so both sides need to find each other. When you want to share or promote the opportunities you are making available, do consider what makes them interesting and then tell people what they will be doing. Just using the word 'volunteer' to describe activities does not convey what volunteers will actually be involved in, leaving questions. How much time can they expect to be involved? Is it regular or a one-off? When putting information together, it is worth considering whether it clearly describes what will be done, outlines the activities and makes the purpose of the activity clear. Setting this out will put the offer into context and explain how being involved will be making a difference. In Practice Example: One, 'A', felt reassured as all that information was provided.

It is also important to consider how we describe an activity, to inspire confidence that volunteering will proactively benefit a cause according to people's circumstances. For some people, using language such as 'need' or 'urgently wanted' can be off-putting. Those who are motivated by building a solution to an immediate need will probably have already started doing something and now look for others to be part of that. Others, may want more assurance regarding the direction being taken, and do not want to be solely relied upon to deliver a solution.

Reflecting about what might put different people off from particular activities gives a chance to try to address potential barriers. People concerned that they do not have the relevant skills may be reassured to see phrases such as 'no experience necessary', 'full training and support giving'. Others might worry that volunteering could be a financial burden, so it may help to let them know 'expenses paid', and to have planned to budget for this. Some people can be intimidated by not seeing any apparent stated ending, as the time to set aside can be a barrier to getting involved in volunteering. In the Community Life Survey 20/21, the main reason for people saying they didn't get involved in volunteering was down to time, either work (48%) or doing other things with their spare time (31%) (Department for Digital, Culture, Media and Sport, 2021). Making clear how much time is expected and for how long can therefore be helpful.

Reaching as many people as possible with the offer of an inclusive volunteering opportunity, requires reflection on how and where to find people, and how to show that the group is welcoming to everyone and keen to build different relationships. Local volunteer centres will be able to help with information about communication and planning for the involvement of different types of local volunteers. People also need to find signing up and getting involved as frictionless and timely as possible. There should be an easy way for a potential volunteer to get in touch and to have a response quickly. Potential volunteers will quickly move on to another opportunity if the process is too long or feels disorganised, no matter how nice a group is or valuable the cause is. There are digital options available to support this, which have become more prevalent during the pandemic and so making communication in this way more likely. We can now reflect on how not being able to get back to someone may mean you lose them.

Practice Example: Two

'B' had recently moved to a new city and was keen to extend his social network by volunteering. He had volunteered before. He wanted to make sure he could do something which was flexible enough to fit in with his busy lifestyle, and had a demonstrable benefit to people, so when he saw a role driving assistance animals to appointments and training centres, he thought it would be ideal. He submitted an application form in September and had an initial reply fairly quickly asking for references. When he received a chasing email about the references, he felt slightly annoyed. He knew they'd been submitted because his referees had shared them with him. But he recognised that these things happened. He heard nothing for a while but was busy anyway so wasn't too bothered but followed up in mid-November only to be told by a coordinator that she was changing jobs and would be handing his case over. 'B' asked if he could have some training dates so he could hold them but again heard nothing back. Four months after his initial application, he received a generic email clearly sent to a range of people asking to state their preferences of times of days so that they could set up something which suited as many of people as possible. 'B' decided that if this was the experience just trying to get on to training for the role, he didn't have much faith for how it would feel actually volunteering, so he decided to withdraw from the process.

5.1.3 Understanding Opportunities and Volunteers

It is important to take time to understand why people want to get involved with the group or cause and the role. Volunteers need to be able to understand what is being looked for and be able to articulate what they are looking for. For many people and activities, this might be about getting to do something quickly then to move on. Often, what is needed just means letting someone know where they have to turn up and who to ask for, such as for a litter pick on the beach. But even here, it is still advisable to factor in time to have a conversation so that both volunteers and volunteer involving organisations can discuss ways to fit the broader requirements with what can be done with a potential volunteer's skills and interests. There could be further opportunities not yet thought of or help that a group wanted where this person might really add value.

It can be daunting for people to put themselves forward as a volunteer, especially if they are not sure what they are getting into, may be worried that they will be letting someone down, or that time expectations could be more than they want or can offer. So providing chances to meet in person or virtually and discuss what they can offer would be helpful. Most people have something to offer and having a chat exploring their interests might help to decide where they could best fit. If, however someone is not suited to what is needed at that time or an organisation cannot meet what someone is looking for, they will need to be told, and be given suggestions for where else they might look. This does not mean competing for volunteers but building a relationship, so it is not losing a volunteer to recommend another group or refer them elsewhere. Perhaps, an identified role can be divided up between different people, each playing to their own strengths and creating a diversity of ideas. So being open to how and where this might be possible can build stronger volunteering relationships in the longer run.

Some activities may require more understanding of a volunteer's attributes and abilities, especially for roles which need softer skills for supporting vulnerable people as with befriending, coaching, leading youth groups. Creating opportunities to let the potential volunteer try out and explore what they might experience can be useful to help them make an informed decision whether they continue.

Here's a chance to reflect on what testing an activity might look like and what you think the pros and cons of such an approach might be.

Practice Example: Three

'C' was very supportive of a local group helping new parents and wanted to give something back to others who had been affected by a similar circumstance. She was very keen to be involved with a new befriending service that was developed. Potential support volunteers are invited to an information session before they formally sign up so that they can have a sense of what kind of calls they might receive and gain an understanding of how they will be expected to respond when hearing particular themes. These sessions can include group conversations on controversial subjects about which a potential volunteer may have strong feelings and is a chance to help them assess whether they'd be able to behave in a way which meets the requirements of the service, such as with neutral empathy. During the information session, she felt quite emotional about one of the topics which was raised and in the follow-up conversation with the session leader afterwards she discussed whether she was ready to follow up at that time. She recognised that she might not be able to support someone appropriately who expressed the views shared during that topic and decided that she wouldn't go through the next stages for that role, but felt privileged to have had the opportunity to try it out and continued volunteering in another capacity for the group.

Providing initial training on what the group is set up to achieve and how a volunteer's involvement will help to do that, is a good opportunity to make people feel comfortable with what's expected of them and reassured that they know what to do. In many cases, this is a good motivator as well, because developing new skills and having different experiences can be a reason for wanting to get involved in volunteering.

As we saw in Practice Example: Three, information sessions are a valuable tool to involve the wider community. In the case of an emotional support helpline, potential volunteers who decide that the role is not for them have been given tools of active listening and a greater understanding of the service which will have positive knock-on effects for the helpline.

Learning doesn't have to be delivered in an old-fashioned, time-intensive 'chalk and talk' training method, and some people may be put off because of associations with school. Sharing learning opportunities are positive, because it's clear that people do learn most through practical experiences while carrying out their role, and offers like peer-peer arrangements will have the twofold effect of creating a welcoming and social atmosphere for a new volunteer and of valuing and developing a more experienced volunteer who can act as a guide.

As well as a generic introduction there will be appropriate specific training for particular aspects of an activity that a volunteer will be doing so that they know what is expected from them and can get started. One of the pieces of information someone is going to need, however casual and low-intensive their role might be, is who their point of contact will be for any queries. Some groups might have the resources to offer a written handbook or guidance for new volunteers. It is helpful to consider having something available for those people who learn best through reflection to refer back to, but this doesn't need to be overcomplicated.

In some cases, people volunteer to use their existing skills so someone could have a lot of relevant experience in the actual task they'll be carrying out, often more than anyone else in the current group, so learning should be adaptable but it is also important that people understand the particularities of any group or organisation.

The time and resource allocated to learning has to be appropriate to the activity. For example, someone at a cheer point for a marathon may only need a quick briefing whereas those who might be visiting people in their homes or rescuing people in danger will need something substantially different. A one size fits all approach to training will not achieve its aims for all and could feel like wasting a volunteer's time. The key element of any initial training is to welcome volunteers, and to let people know the important parts of how they will be involved so that they can start confidently, knowing that they will be supported.

Some people want to volunteer so that they can bring their experience and expertise. Others might get involved because they want to improve their skills or learn something new. Learning and development will continue to be an important contributor to continuing the relationship, not only because it offers ongoing support to a volunteer but also because it shows them that the organisation wants to invest in them. Effective training not only equips people with the confidence and skills to carry out their role, but it also encourages a sense of dedication to it through emphasising their value to the group and the cause.

5.2   Collaborating

Involving volunteers takes time, often money, commitment and other resources. It is worth reflecting on how to maintain a relationship because when it breaks down, the effort of building a relationship has to begin again and existing positive relationships bring others in.

It is just as important to enable an ongoing involvement and keep up their motivations and retain their enthusiasm, and as in any relationship this is something to do with volunteers not to them. People are more likely to want to stay involved if they feel valued and supported. Making sure that a rewarding experience is created will result in not only continuing to involve current motivated volunteers but also means that they will carry positive messages from their volunteering to their broader family, friends and community. So, a volunteer who feels valued and that they're getting something out of it is also a good promoter for a group or cause. This section examines the steps needed to keep people wanting to be involved and will look at:

- Communicating with volunteers,
- Guiding and supporting volunteers,
- Valuing volunteers.

Finding new volunteers is the start of a relationship pathway. Keeping that relationship going is the key to future involvement, which will ultimately ensure that a difference to the people or cause can continue to be made, and improve the offer through being informed by diverse ideas. Focusing as much time on keeping the relationship going with volunteers who are already involved, as giving to building new relationships to involve new volunteers, is crucial and will have knock-on benefits.

Considering how to plan for this ongoing involvement is helpful before starting to connect to volunteers, so resource for support should be in place. Some people only want to come along for one event and may be put off by what they see as constant contact and requests for further help. Before staying in touch with them, organisations will need to have their explicit consent so it is essential to ask for permission and provide clear reasons for doing this. If someone is happy to join an annual guerrilla gardening campaign and doesn't want to receive any other information, they should only be contacted about that event.

Many people want to ensure that they have the chance to feed into the broader strategic development, although others are happier to be directed. It's important to provide an opportunity for this to happen, not only to keep people involved but to keep that opening for shaping new projects which really matter and that might not have been thought of without a broader conversation. Involving volunteers can offer the ability to create solutions which have not been identified before. We're now going to look at how setting up the framework for communicating with volunteers has helped both a volunteering involving organisation and the volunteers.

Practice Example: Four

'D' is a volunteer in a large charity who sent the following message to the volunteer coordinator: "*It's good to hear, too, that feedback from volunteers is not only sought but also acted upon... it really makes a difference to know that our opinions are recognised and valued*".

The charity had found that it was challenging to be able to both communicate with and hear from volunteers but was very keen to be able to offer greater opportunities for volunteers to be involved within its decision-making.

> The charity has developed an active Volunteer Forum, made up of chairs of regional groups representing the geographic areas of the country and bringing together a variety of roles, ranging from fundraising to direct service providers. The forum members are equal participants with staff in developing the volunteering agenda for the charity. And they work with the staff team to review the current state of volunteering within the organisation which then uses this information to develop their strategy.
>
> This was recognised as a powerful incentive for people who volunteered with them.

5.2.1 Communicating

Volunteers want clear information from the group they choose to become involved with, so that they can understand where it's going and how they fit in and it is crucial that they have a voice throughout the organisation. Volunteers are an organisation's key stakeholders. Therefore, planning and resourcing to communicate, so that volunteers receive messages in a consistent way no matter where they are or how they are involved is key. When volunteers are welcomed for the first time, check with them how they want to be updated throughout their time.

Whatever someone's role within a group, everyone wants to recognise that they're part of something larger, and that's where communication comes in. Not only to keep people informed and up-to-date but to be fully involved in consultations regarding the development and future. Creating engaging, welcoming and inclusive communication will help everyone who volunteers, or may be looking at picking up volunteering, to see themselves being involved in that way.

Of course, to be inclusive, communication shouldn't only be coming from one direction in a broadcast manner. So what could be done to proactively listen to volunteers and periodically ask for feedback, either ad hoc or through something more structured, such as in Practice Example: Four. This can help to ensure that volunteers recognise an organisation's vision and also that they can be part of shaping it, which will help them to remain involved and positive, enjoying their role within the group.

Creating a central point or mechanism where key messages can be delivered and having a strategic and transparent and safe way for volunteers to feedback into the organisation will ensure that there's a true user-led or two-way communication, which will help to keep the relationship strong. In Practice Example: Five, we look at what might happen if communications don't achieve what we hope and the chance to keep in touch with each other is missed.

Practice Example: Five

'E' volunteers for a local community helpline providing telephone support to people who had been abused.

Training for the helpline volunteers lasted 4–5 full days before they felt ready to take calls. For the initial calls, a more experienced volunteer would sit in, to be on hand. At the end of every shift, all volunteers were encouraged to debrief if necessary to a more experienced volunteer who had received training in that additional role. Once it was felt that the helpline volunteers had enough experience, this keeping in touch dropped off, although they were offered supervision with counselling students every few months. They were also on shift on their own. Many of the calls which were received were from people who had never declared their abuse before and these were difficult to hear and process; but volunteers felt unwilling to mention that they might want to de-brief as they felt very strongly that they were there for the callers and the organisation needed them to be resilient. The initial training had been excellent and there was enthusiasm and passion for the cause and fondness for the staff at the organisation but very few volunteers were able to give time above a year and the helpline was constantly looking for new volunteers.

5.2.2 Supporting

Taking time to show and offer care, advice and an opportunity to debrief as well as to give and receive feedback can be a key factor in keeping volunteers involved and is indispensable to showing meaningful recognition of volunteer's contribution. Many volunteers want to be sure that there is someone they can go to who will offer support and advice, who will respect their role and their needs. Having regular catchups are also the perfect time to say thank you and learn what keeps people wanting to remain involved, and possibly to address any problems, on either side. As people's motivations change, it's important to understand:

* Why someone volunteered with you in the first place,
* Why they stay involved with you,
* Why those that stop volunteering leave.

Sadly, all too often support sessions are the one area which is overlooked, because of time constraints and conflicting priorities. Being able to keep a volunteer involved through having been able to build up that relationship with them and staying aware of any problems or concerns may well be a better use of time than going through the revolving door of finding new people as others drop out. It could also be ultimately more satisfying and lead to deeper connections, suggestions for alternatives, and more sustainable ways of continuing.

These do need to be relaxed conversations, rather than something which might feel like a paid staff work style appraisal and to be used as an opportunity for two-way feedback. As before, they need to be appropriate to the role, with lighter touch volunteering maybe needing a quick email exchange and offering opportunity to chat and those roles which are more intense and emotional having a broader supervision structure.

Ongoing opportunities for learning and development can also continue to be a good way to support each other, so are there any chances to enable this? There are probably related courses, events and relevant speakers in the area to take part in or collaborate with and the local volunteer centre is likely to have information.

Even very experienced volunteers will benefit from ongoing learning as part of any support offer, hearing from others and sharing good practice, not just to enhance their practice and skills, but also to feel connected to the continuing aims. It's useful to consider how volunteers who have been involved for a time and of course those who have experience in this area, can play a role in developing and delivering any learning and development.

Recognising people's skills and contributions is an important way of showing that they are valued and our next Practice Example looks at how saying thank you need not be flamboyant. How would you would prefer to be noticed and recognised?

Practice Example: Six

'F' volunteers as coach and referee for a small local football club. After the final match of the season, she and the other volunteers who support the events each received a thank you card with a handwritten positive, affirmative message on the back and a packet of sweets. The club held its final matches during Volunteers Week and took the opportunity to recognise the fact that this activity could not happen without the involvement of volunteers providing coaching, scoring, refereeing, event support by posting a double page spread thank you in the programme. 'F' felt that it was these small gestures throughout the year that kept her coming back.

5.2.3 Valuing

Most of us like to be appreciated and recognised for what we've done. This doesn't mean that people are consciously looking for thanks, rather that it becomes noticed if it's never given. Probably, the most important thing that can be done in order to continue a relationship with volunteers is to make sure they know that they and what they do are valued.

Acknowledging the contributions volunteers make is vital, but it's also important to find appropriate ways to do this. For some people, the traditional glitzy awards ceremony is far from motivating and is a real turn off and can feel disproportionate, though others of course love their chance in the limelight and the sense of occasion.

Many organisations have annual Volunteer awards scheme which includes long service certificates and special recognition awards and these can be great social events and also opportunities to involve other members of the community. There are lots of different ways to thank and recognise volunteers but to be really effective these should be tailored. How could volunteers be recognised and rewarded in more personal ways?

Arguably more valuable than the big gestures, such as an award ceremony, are the everyday things that can be done to make volunteers feel valued. We all know that a simple 'thank you' goes a long way. In Practice Example: Six, one of the volunteers told the lead for volunteering that the friendly thanks and ongoing recognition were among the reasons she carried on volunteering. It was simple but effective and this demonstration of success is down to the understanding that the personal relationships built are very important.

The needs of those volunteers who do not respond to an organisation's social events should be taken into consideration when designing engaging plans, which responds to what individuals actually want. Developing ways of saying 'thank you' to volunteers will keep them feeling motivated and valued in a more intrinsic and less tangible way, which becomes embedded in the fabric of volunteering.

The first week of June within the UK is volunteers' week, an occasion for all volunteer involving groups and organisations to showcase and celebrate volunteering in all its forms. This is often marked with thank you cards, social events and some groups send out a news release highlighting the achievement of the volunteers. This offers a positive message demonstrating how what volunteers do is valued as well as showing the range of activities, which could be a useful opportunity to promote a cause and volunteering offers to new people.

While volunteers do not receive any financial reward or payment for their activity, no one should be out of pocket because of their volunteering so it's important to offer expenses for things they may incur as a result of this, such as travelling. It is reasonable to request receipts and advisable to have clear guidance available on what is covered and how to claim. You may find that some volunteers don't want to claim, seeing this as an extra gift to the cause but it's important to offer this option to everyone so as to not inadvertently discriminate against people who may not otherwise be able to afford it.

5.3   Complementing

The elements of volunteering involvement which also need to be considered and factored into your planning because they add value to the experience of becoming and remaining involved are important considerations which stand alongside the volunteer journey but need discrete thought. In this section, we will explore:

- Inclusion
- Problem solving
- Monitoring
- Goodbyes

Practice Example: Seven demonstrates that involving volunteers can support greater inclusiveness within an organisation and that being willing to listen to the needs of volunteers will improve accessibility for all.

> **Practice Example: Seven**
>
> 'G' volunteered to manage the social media account for a region of a charity with a branch network. He had physical disabilities and used a wheelchair and was also very involved with his local Disability network. His role expanded which required more travel across the UK and crucially overnight stays. It became clear that the charity had not fully taken into consideration the needs of wheelchair users into their hotel booking processes, but was open to putting this right. 'G' offered to lead a project looking into this and was given resource of time and people to develop an improvement to the system which was embedded into the charity's ways of working, ultimately benefitting everyone.

5.3.1 Inclusion

One of the strategic reasons for involving volunteers is to enable connection with diverse communities. One of the benefits of volunteering to society as a whole is that people might be more likely to mix with those of different ethnic groups or religious beliefs while volunteering. Nearly 60% of volunteers surveyed for Jump's research 'a bit rich' indicated that they did this (Lawton & Watt, 2019, p. 12).

The key to being able to offer inclusive opportunities is ensuring that those who involve volunteers are supported with the tools and resources to have the confidence and creativity to develop meaningful relationships with different audiences. Part of this is to be clear of the reason why inclusive volunteering is important, and to recognise benefits. Many of the barriers to inclusive volunteering come from existing structures within groups or organisations.

- There may be concern that involving volunteers from different backgrounds or with different characteristics will be more difficult or time-consuming.
- Those wanting to involve volunteers may not feel they have the experience and cultural sensitivity to involve certain groups and are not sure of what to do if issues arise.
- There may be resistance within staff and current volunteer groups to change, either perceived or well founded, especially when they don't feel the need for change, or disagree with the proposed change.

Everyone has biases and we are all products of the world around us and the culture we live in and understanding this and our biases can enable us to counteract those and interrupt them, either as an individual in real time or through changing basic systems and processes in groups or organisations to ensure that we can filter out stereotypes. The most important takeaway is not to make assumptions, but to ask. People are experts in their own conditions and life experiences.

Larger organisations or statutory bodies which may feel further away from the communities with whom they collaborate might want to develop a way to ensure volunteers have a prominent voice, with meaningful involvement of volunteers in governance, service design, quality improvements and professional training. Community groups that are very local might be involved in such ways already, but it can be difficult to remember sometimes to hear from everyone within the movement, so this may well be a relevant reminder.

Much of what we have looked at is with regard to developing clear processes to enable an individual to develop their volunteer involvement in a flexible and supportive way. This will support the move to creating an inclusive culture.

An important question volunteer involving groups need to ask is whether they have created a space for enabling inclusion and involvement. To achieve this, appropriate processes might need to be embedded in existing systems. These give assistance and ensure consideration of planning for diverse groups of volunteers, supporting and enabling those who involve volunteers to feel confident about finding out from a potential volunteer, or from a volunteer whose circumstances have changed, to have conversations regarding their individual needs and how they may be able to adapt, or indeed develop, their involvement.

Key areas to look at are using a structured decision-making process with clear criteria when bringing people in, ensuring meetings are run for full participation and that all contributions are recognised fairly.

It may be helpful to have honest conversations with volunteers and staff who might be finding some of these enhanced processes unnecessary and express doubts as to the importance of encouraging diversity. Review whether there are training needs that could support and overcome any such misunderstanding or concerns.

Motivation is different for everyone and needs to be recognised as such. People from lower social economic groups are likely to have different motivations and needs, compared to what we know about the traditional view of volunteering undertaken by volunteers who have relatively more time and resources. People from higher social economic groups are more likely to cite that they become involved because of personal philosophy or importance of the cause, the elements which we are encouraged to think of as the 'pure' altruistic nature of an ideal volunteer (Lawton & Watt, 2019, p. 9). Linking this to any unconscious bias we may have of what makes an 'ideal volunteer' means we need to be very clear that we are not imbuing any of our messages that volunteering to gain skills, experience or improving social networks is somehow less worthy, and more 'selfish'.

Our next Practice Example looks at what happens when something goes wrong and how ignoring it can make things worse.

Practice Example: Eight

'H' was a volunteer trampolining judge and club committee member. She began volunteering two years ago—partly due to the amount of time she spent at competitions through her daughter's participation as a gymnast but also because she knew that without club officials, the club would not be able to compete at higher level competitions. One Sunday H volunteered to support the club friendly as an official. Based on her past volunteering experience for the club, her expectations were not high; however, on this occasion, even these minimal expectations were not met. For instance, she was not asked if she would like to volunteer, simply told she had been put down to judge; her shift didn't end when it was supposed to and actually overran by two hours; she was expected to help pack away equipment and clear up at the end; she had no time for a lunch break, and even had to buy her own coffee during the day. To add further insult, she wasn't thanked for her contribution and there was no communication afterwards to let her know about the impact that she had made towards fundraising for the club. H shared her annoyance at how she'd been treated and made suggestions about how things could have been better. She didn't receive a response and following another attempt she has now stepped down from the committee and has not judged a competition since.

5.3.2 Problem Solving

There may be times when involving volunteers can have negative consequences and it's important to plan how to address these in advance. Ensuring there's a plan and a process for what to do in case of a complaint is important. Complaints could be from a volunteer, about a volunteer, from a member of the public, from a service user or from a staff member. Having a point of contact to receive these and a clear description of what will happen next will help. Unlike employees, volunteers do not have rights in law. This means that no group or organisation has an obligation to keep a volunteer in a role and it also means that people can stop volunteering whenever they want. However, this does not mean that people who are volunteering can be treated unfairly and there should be procedures in place to support everyone if something does go wrong. In any group, but maybe especially when people are giving time to a cause that feels personally relevant to them, disputes and disagreements may happen. It's important to address these in as timely a manner as possible and aim to resolve them with as little distress to all concerned as possible.

The process should start with simple conversations based on the issue being raised. Hopefully someone being able to feel heard will help to resolve any problem easily. It may, however, be necessary to take this a bit further and make a decision in light of a volunteer's behaviour and whether something should be done to prevent this from affecting the activity being carried out. In some cases, the nature of the concern could be great enough to have to ask the volunteer to step down from their role while it is being looked into.

Concerns need to be treated confidentially and enough time allowed for meetings to discuss issues and possible solutions with those involved. Keeping notes of these meetings is important so that they can be referred to if difficult decisions need to be made. The process should say what potential next steps would be. This might include re-training, offering a different role or in some cases asking a volunteer to leave.

Someone's behaviour can be affected by a variety of factors, either related to their volunteering or outside such as health or personal issues. This may have a bearing on any conversation so acknowledge where things may be going wrong without an automatic assumption of fault. People will probably have said or done things for what they felt were the best reasons so the process should ensure that everyone has the benefit of the doubt and assumes positive intent of all sides. It may be useful to consider how to help the volunteer to organise themselves and take time out.

5.3.3 Monitoring

A basic rule of volunteer involvement should be that it is always of a nature and quality that a volunteer would volunteer again. If involvement practice puts people off volunteering, then it is having a negative impact. We therefore find that a basic rule to assessing quality of an experience is whether a volunteer wants to continue. Of course it cannot wait until a volunteer does no longer want to continue, until we find out something might need changing. That makes it important to monitor the effects of volunteering on the volunteer. This requires understanding how volunteers feel about their involvement, how their contributions are being valued and the satisfaction they feel, or not, about their role and the group or organisation. Gathering information through regular and ongoing monitoring will be helpful and can include:

* Notes from attentive conversations
* Entries in a comment book
* Responses to an annual survey

A great way of feedback is to let volunteers know the results of a survey or share other information from monitoring. Especially for larger programmes or organisations with volunteers involved over a long time, it might be worth considering to monitor levels of well-being which can be compared with the national picture, as available from the Community Life Survey. This is also the time to consider what information to collect on diversity of an organisation's volunteers.

This is much more than about counting numbers and hours. Reducing volunteering to such measures can be counterproductive and is likely to be an unreliable measure of success. It is necessary of course to know about any tasks which may be carried out, to ensure that there is the right amount of people to carry them out and that this can be planned accordingly but the numbers and hours by themselves are not the valuable measure.

Volunteer involvement is based on relationships, and there needs to be the recognition that these can change and sometimes people want to say goodbye. Our next Practice Example looks at this and we'd like you to reflect on what would be an appropriate way to let the relationship end.

Practice Example: Nine

During the COVID-19 pandemic, 'K' was furloughed and with little to do felt increasingly unhappy. His partner forwarded on an email to him with a Facebook link from a group of local residents who supported the local foodbank. They were looking for drivers to take food parcels round while people were asked not to come to the foodbank. 'K' agreed to help out once a week and got to know the other volunteers; including the main organiser of the foodbank whose story was chosen for a special radio programme in June 2021. About a year later once restrictions were lifted and people could start to go to the foodbank themselves, the volunteer drivers were all told that their role was no longer needed, but were encouraged to stay involved. 'K' took this as a reason to decide to leave. The foodbank stays in touch by sending monthly emails, including a recent invitation to summer barbecue, which he deletes unread.

5.3.4 Goodbyes

It may seem counter-intuitive but it's important to consider how to make it easy for people to stop volunteering from the start. People's priorities change during their lives and by recognising that and letting them know they're allowed to leave will give a positive experience that ensures people remain involved and motivated while they are there.

People decide to stop for many reasons. They have too many other commitments, their personal life circumstances change, they're simply not enjoying it anymore. We know that for some years now and as society changes, people are less likely to remain in a particular job or undertake the same hobby or be involved as volunteer in the same way for life. Volunteer involving organisations need to be mindful of this and certainly should not try to manipulate volunteers with moral pressure to stay on. This is likely to cause bad feeling and in any case is against the values of volunteering as set out at the beginning of the book.

Could this be a time to try to capture feedback though? It is a unique opportunity to capture the honest opinions of someone who's been involved with the cause, so is a chance to listen and act on that which is relevant. This also gives an opportunity to enable the volunteer to leave feeling positive, with an experience which will make them into a promoter for the cause and possibly encourage them to return. A leaving pack with a personalised thank you letter, and including an exit survey, is a nice way to show that they're going on a positive note, which might mean they'll come back or recommend volunteering to someone else.

Some people volunteer because it helps them to build skills or experiences for employment or further education. They could be offered a reference which they can use to demonstrate what they've learnt.

People may of course leave because they've been asked to, particularly with regard to problem solving. This should be handled in as empathetic and respectful way as possible.

5.4   Summary and Conclusion

Many organisations and groups don't have the time, skills or capacity to develop the resources which are needed in house. We hope that this chapter has provided a useful overview of key elements to consider. There is a wealth of experience and resources within volunteer involving organisations and volunteering infrastructure organisations that can help people learn key skills. A practical piece of advice for people interested in supporting or learning more about the professional development of those who involve volunteers would be to become themselves involved with existing networks which share resources, information and provide collegial support. This benefits all those who involve volunteers and ultimately the volunteers themselves.

References

Grotz, J., Ledgard, M., & Poland, F. (2020). *Patient and public involvement in health and social care: An introduction to theory and practice.* Imprint Springer Nature and Palgrave Macmillan.

Lawton, R., & Watt, W. (2019). *A Bit Rich: Why is volunteering biased towards higher socio-economic groups* (p. 12). Jump Projects.

6

Summary, conclusion and future prospects

Abstract Chapter Six sums up the previous discussions, considering how awareness of complexity and plurality of thought may affect responses to the changing environment for volunteer involvement. It calls for an open collaborative and respectful conversation about volunteer involvement, including about its negative effects and for reflective volunteer involvement practice to make the relationships on which it is based succeed.

Keywords Discussion · Future · Recommendations

Volunteer involvement requires all concerned thinking and acting together. It is a personal choice which does not necessarily mean asking permission. You can do it on your own initiative, with others or with the support of organisations. Yet, concepts of what is described as volunteer involvement are contested. Furthermore, volunteer involvement and volunteering are not neutral actions. The ways people and organisations seek to involve volunteers are often influenced by individual

J. Grotz and R. Leonard, *Volunteer Involvement*,
https://doi.org/10.1007/978-3-031-19221-0_6

and political ideologies. There is no single agreed concept of volunteer involvement or broad agreement of how to involve and be involved in practice. Any suggestion that there is only one way, or any descriptions that exclude particular types of volunteer involvement, rather than capture its breadth, should be treated with great caution and reflectively interrogated as to who and what may be excluded and the reasons why.

We hope that in the previous chapters, we have offered the broad background and presented a balanced picture, to encourage thinking and acting together, collaboratively and respectfully, for everyone who wants to involve volunteers, for policymakers, funders and all those with a role to play. We hope that the exercises have helped you to critically reflect on, to ponder and learn from volunteer involvement, with kind curiosity, informing your future actions, practice, policies and funding decisions. Making such connections can relate to the future of volunteer involvement, allowing to explore further complexity, plurality, diversity and relationships, and to support reflection.

6.1   An Example of Our Humanity

The impulse to do something which makes a difference to others, without being forced to do so, and without expecting financial or other direct, concrete rewards, we believe is something uniquely human and universal. There can be no doubt that volunteer involvement is happening in all parts of society, every day, around the globe and we can be confident that volunteer involvement will continue, morphing into other, new and old, different and similar types of volunteer involvement, vividly seen in many examples of community responses to the COVID-19 pandemic, as illustrated here:

> 41% of the thousands of Facebook groups formed in March 2020 specifically to support neighbours through the first lockdown are still going strong 25 months on. With far fewer people self-isolating or requiring Covid-specific support, the activity of these groups has moved on to a whole range of other issues including community kitchens, skills exchanges and even housebuilding. (We are right here 2022)

The role of volunteer involvement in societies will also keep changing, as with 'building equal and inclusive societies', which has been recognised in 2022 State of the World's Volunteerism Report (United Nations Volunteers Programme, 2021). Furthermore, the way volunteers got involved during the COVID-19 pandemic has also triggered new conversations raising concerns that the more structured forms of volunteering such as through charities are attracting fewer volunteers.

> Volunteer rates have struggled to recover in the aftermath of past periods of collective difficulty, and the onset of an unprecedented squeeze on family incomes is only likely to make it harder to return to pre-pandemic volunteer levels. (Matt Whittaker of Pro Bono Economics quoted in Ricketts 2022)

In England, officially counted numbers of volunteers have fallen over the last 20 years, despite high profile events such as the London Olympic and Paralympics, leading to more calls to raise efforts to promote awareness of how volunteering is an integral part of our social fabric.

> We want a future in which a culture of volunteering is further ingrained in the collective psyche, part of everyone's life, from childhood to later life, and woven into the activities and pastimes of day-to-day living. (Vision for Volunteering 2022)

Given that most people (70%) in the NCVO Time Well Spent survey (McGarvey et al., 2019a, p. 47) reported not having accessed services provided by volunteers in the preceding year seems to demonstrate that even when primed to discuss volunteering, people are just not aware of the full range of volunteering roles and actions, nor that it is highly likely that they have actually interacted with a volunteer, or when this was. The report does seem to confirm a lack of wider social recognition of volunteers and the activities they undertake.

Yet, as well as needing more awareness of the act of volunteering itself, understanding its complexities through more promotion and better explanation might also be needed. Volunteering is already ever-present in people's lives, both as so many people act as volunteers and interact with someone who is volunteering, even if they don't recognise it as such. This might be because volunteering is described in a multitude of ways and manifests in different forms, from duty and service reflected in Beveridge's 'philanthropic motive', to mutual aid, leisure, campaigning and more. These different forms may not always be recognised or respected in the same way. Ensuring debates on volunteering are more inclusive, might help to focus understanding and attention on its range and value.

The description of 'volunteering' in this book encapsulates the widest possible context, not restricting it to particular areas. It captures the activities undertaken through organisations and those that are not, as long as the activities reflect the three core components 'choice', 'not predominantly for money', 'making a difference' and include the restriction to 'outside one's own family'. Maybe, most importantly, this description of volunteering recognises that people are different, that they can choose to have different roles, that they change and that they are not to be 'used' or 'made to fit' within existing opportunities or programmes.

Involving volunteers is likely to be a valuable and meaningful way of addressing some of society's larger problems, but that can never be its sole purpose and it is definitely not an easy, quick or cheap fix. Neither is it an end in itself. Rather volunteer involvement is a powerful way of achieving people's own choices, and is an act of democracy. The most effective way of raising awareness and possibly involving more people better, is to be informed by volunteers, not just by those organisations which seek to involve them. Policymakers should factor this into their planning and build in mechanisms to empower volunteers, making sure that volunteers are involved in decisions that affect them. A volunteer put it this way: *"Worst experience of being a volunteer is when decisions that affect your work are taken by people in positions of authority without consultation"* (Grotz et al., 2022). While Scotland's Volunteering Action Plan 2022, looks at the importance of voice, which is linked to power:

> Build Voice capacity through embedding Voice (especially volunteers' voice) into key decision-making structures and building 'voice gathering' capacity (developing skills, educating and providing guides for individuals and organisations). (Scottish Government 2022, p. 15)

6.2   Conceived of in Many Different Ways

We know that people think about volunteering in diverse ways, organise it differently, influenced by their broader worldview. Volunteering does not just take place within formally constituted organisations with people carrying out pre-defined activities in a transactional manner but also includes someone fly-posting a QR code to invite others to a 'sit-in' protest or a neighbourhood organising a street party.

It is worth noting that despite the apparent downturn in people volunteering through traditional models by 2021, there was an increase in people volunteering not through a group, with 33% of people saying they had volunteered on a monthly basis (Department for Digital, Culture, Media and Sport, 2021). This is unsurprising in the context of COVID-19, as we also saw in Chapter 2 that people will come together to help during crises. "*Informal voluntary action, in the form of individuals and emergent groups, is an important resource and capacity for emergency response*" (Twigg & Mosel, 2017, p. 443). However, it is also indicative of possible change.

This plurality of thought can be seen as a major strength of volunteer involvement and should be actively embraced. If volunteer involvement is solely discussed in terms of human resources management, this assumes all power lies within organisations and would move volunteering away from individual agency, people's motivations and interests, and power to act on them. Planning for, recognising and allowing for spontaneous and more fluid volunteering will ensure that more volunteers can enjoy a better experience and are able to make the difference they want. The approach to practice highlighted in this book is as valid for involving mostly self-directed volunteers, as for people who would prefer to be involved via a more traditional transactional route. Volunteer-led groups value how they can develop in a relaxed free-flowing way, with evidence that they would feel *"strongly that imposing more formal systems of volunteer management on them would be inappropriate and ineffective"* (Ockenden & Hutin, 2008, p. 35). However, volunteer-led groups are not immune to challenges of sharing power, though it may appear more visible within staff-led organisations and there is plenty of space to learn and share across different forms of volunteering and groups which involve them.

> Volunteering can be a driving force in creating a fairer and more equitable society. This will require us to tackle power imbalances across society— imbalances which, at their root, are about the relationships between organisations, communities and individuals. We believe that to create thriving communities requires power to be devolved—from the state to communities, from organisations to individuals. (Vision for Volunteering 2022)

It must be said, however, that plurality is not always welcome. It remains a challenge to recognise that concepts of volunteering are based on ideologies and that this impacts on making decisions regarding which volunteering activities are encouraged and supported. Recognising ideologies challenges the status quo and those driving single issues, as well as questioning entrenched views on volunteer involvement as service.

Understanding and embracing plurality, and respecting others' diverse views, can enable us to judge, not just where specific involvement activities are located in the complex landscape of volunteering, but also to assess the various interests and views of everyone involved, and how these affect volunteer involvement practices. As before and always, such reflection may best be done together with volunteers.

6.3   Not Always an Inherently Good Thing

It is simply inconceivable that an activity as broad as volunteer involvement is only beneficial. We hope that in the future, we can talk more openly about all sides of volunteering, good, bad and indifferent. Openly sharing information not just celebrating successes but also learning from challenges and mistakes, from misconduct or other negative sides of volunteering, would be a good start.

Volunteering is known to have benefits to volunteers, including individual well-being, but it seems as though those who would receive the greatest benefit from volunteering may also be those who are least likely to get involved and so to reap them (Stuart et al., 2020). Therefore future conversations might consider articulating where the positive effects of volunteering may not be reaching those most likely to benefit. It is also important to understand and respond to some of the negative views of volunteering. Not doing so could make it more challenging to create a fully inclusive culture or offer, where people with different views can also be heard.

As in questions regarding plurality of thought, acknowledging and engaging with the challenges of volunteer involvement might lead to more inclusive volunteering. To understand and overcome inequity, we need constant and deliberate efforts consistently capturing and hearing the experiences of people who have found it hard to participate in volunteering or to do so without experiencing discrimination. Acting on feedback will enable volunteer involvement to continuously improve, developing appropriate safeguards and leading to a more egalitarian volunteer experiences.

Finally, not telling the full story of volunteer involvement, in the worst cases gas lighting, making people feel in the wrong if they have negative experiences, may fatally diminish credibility.

6.4   Based on Relationships

It may well be wise to be suspicious of any plans to involve 'armies' of volunteers. Armies dress the same and follow orders. Volunteers are different and the places where and the ways they become involved are different. Volunteer involvement concerns respectful relationships between key players from large to small organisations, policymakers and funders, volunteers and those involving them. Responsibilities cannot be left as an incidental add-on for someone with no skills or interest in actively doing this. Howlett's paper on developing volunteer management as a profession, cites Julia Neuberger, the chair of the Commission on the Future of Volunteering 2007 as suggesting that this role *"was so important that people should not be promoted to senior management posts unless they had been volunteer organisers at some point in their career"* (Howlett, 2010, p. 358).

Viewing volunteers as 'resources' which are 'owned' by particular organisations may cause a problem as people follow their enthusiasm for a given cause across boundaries. Those involving volunteers must recognise people as free to move across organisations, groups and sectors and that the role of those who involve volunteers is to enable this rather than obstruct or manipulate out of competitiveness. The more effortless the experience of volunteers, the more likely will be collaboration and relationship building between all relevant bodies.

Given such diversity, volunteer involvement needs to be personal and aligned to what individuals want to do and to get out of it, not just concerned with filling vacant volunteer roles. Involving volunteers helps creating and enabling collaborative opportunities. If these broader needs of volunteers are not met, they may move away to seek other ways to meet their personal goals and motivations and so remove chances of more informed solutions to a problem a group wants to address.

Starting with building relationships, not filling role descriptions, as the cornerstone of volunteer involvement can help this. Seeing each other as composed of various interests will help to create links and connections. Having a prepared profile might be useful in a conversation, recognising that some people will want clear boundaries, however, this is also the opportunity to collaboratively develop and share what can be done and to begin a relationship, rather than just giving instructions. One of the themes from Scotland's Volunteering Action Plan (Scottish Government, 2022) is relationship building:

> actions have identified where relationships must be strong or strengthened; between 'volunteering' and 'community engagement' partners; and between national and local stakeholders. (p. 23)

Groups and organisations which involve volunteers can collaborate to develop good relationships themselves rather than creating competition between them and jointly share resources to enable good volunteer involvement. This ultimately gives an improved experience to volunteers and should also include ensuring that the volunteer's voices are heard.

6.5   Reflective Volunteer Involvement

During the COVID-19 pandemic, people and agencies collaborated overnight in ways they had often not done before. The pandemic put a spotlight on how volunteer involvement is diverse and multilayered. Rulebooks were thrown away (Meakin & Grotz, 2020). As some now reach again for the old 'how to' guidebooks, 'Vision for Volunteering', is seeking flexibility and learning, and calls for 'experimentation' instead.

> We want experimentation, learning and flexibility to be a natural, constant part of volunteering, not just a temporary bolt-on in times of crisis or Covid. (Vision for Volunteering 2022)

Reflecting on volunteer involvement, remaining curious, challenging our own and others' assumptions and thoughts and taking interest in why others may have different views can help to better experiment. The basic premise of an experiment is that we don't know exactly what will happen, and that it might not go the way we hope it will. This is not failing but learning. All of us, who want to involve volunteers, need to fully understand what volunteering encompasses and to critically reflect on our practice.

> Learning is Essential to Developing Ourselves, Our Organisations, Our Local communities and the issues we care most about. Learning together and learning with one another helps build deeper, more trusting relationships.....While learning is a mutually reinforcing activity it can also be a luxury—we're often too busy 'delivering' to invest appropriate time and 'space' to learn. (Scottish Government, 2022, p. 16)

Measuring the outcomes we hope to achieve, might help us improve. Involving volunteers in evaluations means they can judge and see the value of their involvement and the result in volunteers being supported as inclusively and easily as possible. This is as important within a wholly volunteer-led group as within an organisation with a staff team.

6.6   Concluding Thoughts

Money cannot buy what volunteer involvement offers because it is not done for money. However, financial investment to support volunteer involvement is needed in some areas. But maybe even more importantly, being open to explore not just its full potential but also its real and persistent challenges, might bring more social, cultural, physical and economic value than policymakers dare to believe.

As we look into the future, it seems clear that people remain committed to volunteer involvement. However, the ways volunteers are involved will naturally change. Some might be planned, some just happening. As we hear from 'Vision for Volunteering' in England, the Scottish Government and from the United Nations, developing models of volunteer involvement may be less likely to suit the current prevailing set-up found in many volunteer involving organisations, and in much current thinking on responses to volunteer involvement as people management. New ways of providing support, rather than seeking easy fixes to problems not caused by volunteers or volunteer involvement, are likely to be based on where people themselves are, enabling volunteers to bring their own power and strengths to solutions.

Our intention here is to help you, the reader, to recognise and successfully negotiate tensions and challenges inherent in ensuring that volunteer involvement experiences can be positive. We have sought to encourage you to critically assess approaches you encounter and to consider how to enrich volunteer involvement and to be more responsive to the societal challenges ahead facing all of us.

When considering the future of volunteer involvement, we therefore recommend concentrating on:

* creating awareness of complexity by recognising that people are different and have agency, rather than compartmentalising volunteering activities and trying to fit volunteers into pre-set activities,
* actively embracing plurality of thought in volunteer involvement, rather than sticking to single models,

- recognising all features of volunteer involvement, good, bad and indifferent, rather than looking solely for benefits and ignoring concerns being raised,
- speaking of relationships, rather than armies and volunteer numbers and volunteering hours
- and encouraging ongoing reflection, rather than creating more abstract and wordy toolkits and rule books.

It cannot be said often enough, that if volunteer involvement is not at least a little bit enjoyable, people will not do it for long. Volunteering is undertaken by people coming together to make a difference, sometimes in quite difficult circumstances. Being interested in others and building meaningful and ongoing relationships must therefore be integral to the practice of volunteer involvement. We hope that you have found enjoyment in reading the book, reflecting on some of our questions and challenges for you, and even in disagreeing with us!

We hope you will take from this book that kind curiosity should underpin volunteer involvement theory and that conviviality, respect and enjoyment should be integral to the practice of volunteer involvement.

References

Department for Digital, Culture, Media and Sport. (2021). *Community Life Survey 2020/21*. Report on the webpages of the Department for Digital, Culture, Media and Sport. https://www.gov.uk/government/statistics/community-life-survey-202021. Accessed 27 August 2022.

Grotz, J., Connolly, S., Woodard, R., and Parkinson, E. (2022) *Volunteering Voices: A future vision for Hastings*, Norwich: Institute for Volunteering Research.

Howlett, S. (2010). Developing volunteer management as a profession. *Voluntary Sector Review, 1*(3), 355–360.

McGarvey, A., Jochum, V., Davies, J., Dobbs, J., & Hornung, L. (2019a). *Time well spent: A national survey on the volunteer experience*. NCVO.

Meakin, B., & Grotz, J. (2020). *Throwing away the rulebook: Five things you should consider when planning interactive online events, to make them more inclusive.* Blog on the webpages of the Applied Research Collaboration East of England. https://arc-eoe.nihr.ac.uk/node/271. Accessed 27 August 2022.

Ockenden, N., & Hutin, M. (2008). *Volunteering to lead: A study of leadership in small volunteer led groups IVR 2008* (p. 35). Institute for Volunteering Research.

Scottish Government. (2022). *Scotland's volunteering action plan.* Scottish Government. https://www.gov.scot/publications/scotlands-volunteering-action-plan/. Accessed 26 July 2022.

Stuart, J., Kamerāde, D., Connolly, S., Ellis Paine, A., Nichols, G., & Grotz, J. (2020). *The impacts of volunteering on the subjective wellbeing of volunteers: A rapid evidence assessment.* London: What Works Centre for Wellbeing and Spirit of 2012. https://whatworkswellbeing.org/wp-content/uploads/2020/10/Volunteer-wellbeing-technical-report-Oct2020-a.pdf. Accessed 31 May 2022.

Twigg, J., & Mosel, I. (2017). Emergent groups and spontaneous volunteers in urban disaster response. *Environment and Urbanization, 29*(2), 443–458. https://doi.org/10.1177/0956247817721413. https://journals.sagepub.com/doi/full/10.1177/0956247817721413. Accessed 28 June 2022.

United Nations Volunteers (UNV) Programme. (2021). *2022 state of the world's volunteerism report. Building equal and inclusive societies.* United Nations Volunteers (UNV) programme.

Glossary

Agency: 'Agency' describes an individual's will, intent, and determination and power to act on it. In this book, we refer to agency to describe how a volunteer chooses, or feels able to choose their involvement. Some people want to shape the whole experience and others want to be directed. Both are valid. Not all people have the same level of agency.

Assets: 'Assets' describes the collective resources which communities and individuals have at their disposal to develop solutions, such as skills, buildings, spaces, connection, experience and passion. The term is often used in approaches viewing individuals and communities through the lens of the assets which they have, rather than the problems or needs they may have are transformative and volunteering is a powerful way of sharing assets.

AVM: 'AVM' stands for Association of Volunteer Managers. AVM is an independent membership body that aims to support, represent and champion people in volunteer management in the UK regardless of field, discipline or sector. It has been set up by and for people who manage volunteers.

Beneficiaries: 'Beneficiaries' describes people who receive support, in this book, from volunteers, albeit volunteers can also be beneficiaries.

J. Grotz and R. Leonard, *Volunteer Involvement*, https://doi.org/10.1007/978-3-031-19221-0

Benefit: 'Benefit' generally describes something that produces results intended to have positive effects. We do not use the word in our definition of volunteering because people don't agree on what can be a positive result and also because we believe its inclusion may lead to a bias in positive reporting.

Branch: 'Branch' describes one of the offices or groups which forms part of a larger organisation. These are separated but accountable to the central office. Several large UK charities have a network of branches, many of which are entirely volunteer-led. In some cases, branches may be separate charitable entities and linked within a federated structure.

Cause: 'Cause' describes a principle, aim, movement or goal in which an individual or group is interested and to which they are dedicated to supporting and reaching. As we have seen in Chapter One, 'the cause was important to me' is one of the main reasons people have said that they get involved in volunteering. Causes can be opposing such as an example we use in Chapter Three of disabled anglers and anti-angling saboteurs.

Charity: 'Charity' describes an organisation which is legally constituted to provide or facilitate help and support for a specific cause and to those who need it. Charities' profits go towards achieving their defined aims and objectives.

Choice: 'Choice' describes that capacity to choose. It is one of the core principles of volunteer involvement.

Community: 'Community' is a complex and contested term which generally requires context such as geography, ethnicity or shared experience, interest or work practice. Community means different things to different people at different times.

DBS: 'DBS' stands for Disclosure and Barring Service. A DBS check is free for volunteers. A DBS check will contain details of both spent and unspent convictions, cautions, reprimands and warnings that are held on the Police National Computer, which are not subject to filtering. This service covers England, Wales, Channel Islands and Isle of Man and within Northern Ireland is operated by Access NI. An enhanced DBS check is suitable for people working with children or adults in certain circumstances such as those in receipt of health care or personal care.

Engagement: 'Engagement' is also a complex and contested term. We have used it within the book to describe the strength of a volunteer's connection to the group or cause with which they are involved, to understand how they feel about their involvement. However, organisations have also used the term as a synonym for 'involvement' and 'participation'.

ESV: 'ESV' stands for Employer Supported Volunteering. ESV provides employees the opportunity to volunteer with support from their employer, whether this is in the form of time off for individual volunteering or in a programme developed by the employer such as a team challenge event or ongoing arrangement with a community partner.

Evaluation: 'Evaluation' in this book describes the systematic assessment of the quality of outcomes of activities, projects or programmes, including volunteer involvement.

Ideology: 'Ideology' describes a set of beliefs and ideas upon which opinions are made, a manner or content of thinking which shapes the way an individual or group thinks or operates.

Impact: 'Impact' is a term used in many policy and funding documents to identify the overarching difference a programme or activity makes.

Inclusion: 'Inclusion' describes creating an environment where everybody is treated fairly and equally as distinct individuals, have a sense of belonging, feel respected and valued, seen for who they are and not experience discriminatory action.

Infrastructure: 'Infrastructure' in this book describes the basic physical and organisational structures needed for the operation of a network, such as to enable volunteering in a particular area.

Involvement: 'Involvement' is also a contested term. It describes enabling others to take part in an activity, in this case volunteering. Within this book, we have used this term to describe how to enable volunteers to contribute, ensuring that people are part of developing the solutions and is done with rather than to those taking part.

IVR: 'IVR' stands for Institute for Volunteering Research. IVR is a Research Institute at the University of East Anglia. It was set up in 1997 to undertake high-quality research on volunteering.

Management (volunteer): 'Management' in this book describes volunteer involvement akin to HR practices. We deliberately didn't want to use that term in this book with regard to volunteering but recognise that the term volunteer management is used to describe the roles, particularly for paid staff, of enabling volunteering.

Misconduct: 'Misconduct' describes behaviour not conforming to prevailing standards or rules. In Chapter Three, we look at misconduct by volunteers and by volunteer involving organisations and also at where volunteering activities are deliberate transgressions as protests.

NAVCA: 'NAVCA' stands for National Association for Voluntary and Community Action. NAVCA is a national membership body for local support and development organisations in England.

NCADC: 'NCADC' stands for National Coalition of Anti-Deportation Campaigns now called 'Right to Remain'. 'Right to Remain' is a registered charity working with communities, groups and organisations across the UK to assist people who leave their homes fleeing war, persecution and poverty.

NCS: 'NCS' stands for National Citizen Service. NCS is a voluntary personal and social development programme for 15–17 year olds in England and Northern Ireland, funded largely by money from the UK Government. As part of the programme, the young people volunteer.

NCVO: 'NCVO' stands for National Council for Voluntary Organisations. NCVO is an umbrella body for voluntary and community organisations in England.

NHS: 'NHS' stands for National Health Service. NHS England is the publicly funded healthcare system in England. Scotland, Wales and Northern Ireland also have an NHS.

Outcomes: 'Outcomes' describes the changes a project or initiative is designed to deliver. In this book, it is used as part of a 'logic framework'.

Outputs: 'Output' describes the direct results or products of a project or initiative. In this book, it is used as part of a 'logic framework'.

Participatory model: 'Participatory model' describes volunteer involvement mostly linked to 'mutual aid', 'leisure', 'democracy' and 'campaigning' like sharing personal problems and participating in therapeutic interventions. It can be observed commonly in associations which are run entirely by volunteers and relate more to mutual benefits, such as, in self-help groups.

Participation: 'Participation' is a term used sometimes interchangeably with 'involvement' or 'engagement' by various organisations. In this book, it is only used in particular contexts, for example, in Chapter Two, about how volunteering is conceived.

Power: 'Power' in this book describes the ability of individuals or groups to have capacity and capability to act in a certain way. This has links to the use of agency and assets.

PSV: 'PSV' stands for Police Support Volunteers. PSVs volunteer for the Police for example at police station front counters, undertaking general administration, vehicle maintenance, criminal investigation support, updating victims and witnesses, CCTV monitoring.

PVG: 'PVG' stands for Protecting Vulnerable Groups Scheme. PVG is managed by Disclosure Scotland ensuring people who are unsuitable to work with children and protected adults cannot do regulated work with these vulnerable groups.

RNLI: RNLI stands for Royal National Lifeboat Institution. RNLI saves lives at sea around the coasts of the United Kingdom, the Republic of Ireland, the Channel Islands and the Isle of Man, as well as on some inland waterways.

RSPB: 'RSPB' stands for Royal Society for the Protection of Birds. RSPB protect bird's habitats, save species and seek to end the nature and climate emergency.

Service users: 'Service User' is a contested term describing people who are in receipt of or affected by services including in the case of volunteer involvement those offered by and supported by volunteers.

Stakeholder(s): 'Stakeholder'(s) describes anyone who may in any way be affected by or interested in the work of an organisation or project. The way in which the term is used varies with the organisation and the context and it is best practice to check who it includes. In addition, projects or organisations may need to regularly assess who their stakeholders are, what role they may play and how the project or organisation addresses their needs.

Statutory organisation(s): 'Statutory organisation(s)' describes organisations established by Acts of Parliament in the UK, or other legislating bodies in other countries, often providing services paid for by the government such as the NHS and Local Authorities but also organisations which have duties to inspect or audit them, such as the Audit Commission or the Charity Commission.

Social capital: 'Social capital' describes the networks of relationships among people who live and work in a particular community which makes that community function well and the impact that relationships have on the resources within the community and larger society.

Staff (paid): 'Staff' describes someone who is under contractual obligation to provide work for an organisation for payment and other employment rights. In this book, we deliberately distinguish between staff and volunteers, and the activities they undertake, describing staff activities as work, and volunteer activities as volunteering.

Theory of change: 'Theory of change' describes a range of approaches to evaluating impact.

Transgressive: 'Transgressive' describes activities with purposes that do not conform with prevailing standards or laws, or where the purpose of the activity does not conform with prevailing standards or laws.

Transactional model: 'Transactional model' describes volunteer involvement mostly linked to the type 'philanthropic' or 'service', volunteering for others, like meeting a need by helping to deliver services. Volunteering within this model takes place most commonly within the large, volunteer involving organisations run by paid staff.

TUC: 'TUC' stands for Trades Union Congress. TUC is a federation of trade unions in England and Wales.

VCSE: 'VCSE' stands for Voluntary, Community and Social Enterprise. This term, often used interchangeably with 'third sector' or 'voluntary and community sector', has no clearly agreed definition. It usually describes any organisation, whether or not incorporated, that operates for a social purpose. It generally includes charities; a wide range of enterprises operating for primarily social purposes, including co-operatives or community interest companies, and all forms of unincorporated associations.

Volunteering: 'Volunteering' is a contested term which we explain in this book. We use the following definition: *Volunteering is an individual's activity undertaken by choice, without concern for financial gain and intended to make a difference outside one's own family.*

Volunteering, formal: 'Volunteering (formal)' usually describes volunteering through organisations such as clubs or charities to distinguish from other forms of volunteering. It is often associated with specific volunteer roles, set hours and may involve forms of supervision. We deliberately do not use the term in this book other than in specific contexts.

Volunteering, informal: 'Volunteering (informal)' usually describes volunteering arranged by volunteers themselves. It can include helping neighbours or participating in social action. We deliberately do not use the term in this book other than in specific contexts.

WCVA: 'WCVA' stands for Wales Council for Voluntary Action. WCVA is a national membership organisation for voluntary organisations in Wales.

References

Abel-Smith, B. (1964). *The hospitals 1800–1948*. Heinemann.

Action Together. (2022). *What is a mutual aid group?* Explanation on Action Together webpages for Oldham, Rochdale and Tameside. https://www.act iontogether.org.uk/mutual-aid#1. Accessed 27 August 2022.

ACT UP London. (2022). *About*. Introduction on webpages of ACT UP London. https://actuplondon.wordpress.com/about/. Accessed 27 August 2022.

Age UK. (2021). *Helping the older people who need us the most, a pandemic year—Rising to the challenge: Age UK Report of Trustees and Annual Accounts 2020/21*. Age UK. https://www.ageuk.org.uk/globalassets/age-uk/docume nts/annual-reports-and-reviews/age-uk-annual-report-2021.pdf. Accessed 26 June 2022.

Aguirre, B. E., Macias-Medrano, J., Batista-Silva, J. L., Chikoto, G. L., Jett, Q. R., & Jones-Lungo, K. (2016). Spontaneous volunteering in emergencies. In D. H. Smith, R. A. Stebbins, & J. Grotz (Eds.), *The Palgrave handbook of volunteering, civic participation, and nonprofit associations* (Vol. 1, pp. 311–329). Palgrave Macmillan.

Aldrich, D. P., & Crook, K. (2008). Strong civil society as a double-edged sword: Siting trailers in post-Katrina New Orleans. *Political Research Quarterly, 61*(3), 379–389.

© The Author(s), under exclusive license to Springer Nature Switzerland AG 2022
J. Grotz and R. Leonard, *Volunteer Involvement*,
https://doi.org/10.1007/978-3-031-19221-0

Almond, P., Bates, A., & Wilson, C. (2015). Circles of support and accountability: Criminal justice volunteers as the 'deliberative public.' *The British Journal of Community Justice, 13*(1), 25–40.

Amnesty International. (2022). *Together we are powerful.* Page on the website of Amnesty International. https://www.amnesty.org/en/get-involved/. Accessed 27 June 2022.

Association of Volunteer Managers. (2022). *About us.* Page on the website of the Association of Volunteer Managers. https://volunteermanagers.org.uk/about/. Accessed 27 August 2022.

Aves, G. (1969). *The voluntary worker in social services: Report of a Committee Jointly set up by the Council for Social Service and the National Institute for Social Work Training.* Bedford Square Press and George Allen & Unwin.

Barker, P. (2016). *Philip Barker: 1866 and all that.* A blog on the website Inside the Games. https://www.insidethegames.biz/articles/1040094/philip-barker-1866-and-all-that. Accessed 27 August 2022.

Beresford, P. (2021). *Participatory ideology: From exclusion to involvement.* Policy Press.

Beveridge, L. (1948). *Voluntary action.* George Allen & Unwin.

Black Lives Matter. (2022). *About.* Page on the website of Black Lives Matter. https://blacklivesmatter.com/about/. Accessed 27 June 2022.

Bluebell Railway. (2021). *Trust & society combined report & accounts 2021.* Bluebell Railway. https://www.bluebell-railway.co.uk/bluebell/soc/notices/trust_brps_accounts_only.pdf. Accessed 27 June 2022.

Bluebell Railway. (2022). *Volunteer at Bluebell Railway.* Page on the Bluebell Railway website. https://www.bluebell-railway.com/volunteer-at-bluebell-railway/. Accessed 27 June 2022.

Borkman, T. (1999). *Understanding self-help/mutual aid: Experiential learning in the commons.* Rutgers University Press.

Bourdillon, A. F. C. (1945). *Voluntary social services: Their place in the modern state.* Methuen & Co Ltd.

Brewis, G., Russell, J., & Holdworth, C. (2010). *Bursting the bubble: Students, volunteering, and the community, full report.* Institute for Volunteering, Research and National Co-ordination Centre for Public Engagement.

British Disabled Angling Association. (2021). *Report of the trustees and unaudited financial statements for the year ended 30 June 2021.* British Disabled Angling Association.

British Red Cross. (2021). *Trustees' report and accounts.* British Red Cross. https://www.redcross.org.uk/about-us/how-we-are-run/our-finances/annual-reports-and-accounts. Accessed 26 June 2022.

Brodie, E., Hughes, T., Jochum, V., Miller, S., Ockenden, N., & Warburton, D. (2011). *Pathways through participation: What creates and sustains active citizenship?* NCVO, IVR, involve. https://involve.org.uk/resources/public ations/project-reports/pathways-through-participation. Accessed 27 August 2022.

Bryant, R. A., & Harvey, A. G. (1996). Posttraumatic stress reactions in volunteer fire fighters. *Journal of Traumatic Stress, 9*(1), 51–62.

Centre for Ageing Better. (2020). *Helping out: Taking an inclusive approach to engaging older volunteers.* Centre for Aging Better. https://ageing-better.org. uk/sites/default/files/2021-08/Helping-out-engaging-older-volunteers.pdf. Accessed 26 June 2022.

Charity Commission. (2022). *Charities in England and Wales—27 August 2022.* Information on the website of the Charity Commission. https://register-of-charities.charitycommission.gov.uk/sector-data/sector-overview. Accessed 27 August 2022.

Chartered Institute of Personnel and Development. (2015). *On the brink of a game-changer? Building sustainable partnerships between companies and voluntary organisations.* Chartered Institute of Personnel and Development, IVR. https://www.cipd.co.uk/Images/on-brink-game-changer_2015_tcm18-9047.pdf. Accessed 27 August 2022.

Church of England. (2022). *Managing volunteers.* Webpage on the Church of England website. https://www.churchofengland.org/resources/commun ity-action/managing-volunteers. Accessed 26 June 2022.

Citizens Advice. (2022). *Volunteering with citizens advice.* Page on the website of Citizens Advice. https://www.citizensadvice.org.uk/about-us/support-us/ volunteering/. Accessed 27 June 2022.

Cnaan, R., Handy, F., & Wadsworth, M. (1996). Defining who is a volunteer: Conceptional and empirical considerations. *Nonprofit and Voluntary Sector Quarterly, 23*, 335–351.

Commission of the European Communities. (2004). *SEC(2004) 628 commis-sion staff working paper—Analysis of the replies of the Member States of the European Union and the acceding countries to the Commission ques-tionnaire on voluntary activities of young people.* Commission of the Euro-pean Communities. http://ec.europa.eu/youth/archive/whitepaper/post-lau nch/sec(2004)628_en.pdf. Accessed 16 March 2010.

Commission on the Future of the Voluntary Sector. (1996). *Meeting the challenge of change: Voluntary action into the 21st century.* NCVO.

Commission on the Future of Volunteering. (2008). *Report of the commission on the future of volunteering and manifesto for change.* Volunteering England.

Community Trade Union. (2021). *What is a trade union.* Page on the website of Community Trade Union last updated 15 November 2021. https://community-tu.org/who-we-are/what-is-a-trade-union/. Accessed 27 June 2022.

Connolly, S., & Woodard, R. (2022). *The value of values: Calculating the economic and individual benefits of workplace volunteering.* Blog on the website of the Institute for Volunteering Research. https://www.uea.ac.uk/web/groups-and-centres/institute-for-volunteering-research/blog. Accessed 27 August 2022.

Conservation Volunteers. (2020). *For people and green spaces: A thriving network for everyone: Strategy 2021–25.* The Conservation Volunteers. https://www.tcv.org.uk/wp-content/uploads/2021/07/Strategy_brochure_visual-final-singles.pdf. Accessed 27 June 2022.

Conservative Party. (2008). *A stronger society: Voluntary action in the 21st century, responsibility agenda* (Policy Green paper No. 5). London: Conservative Party. http://www.conservatives.com/~/media/Files/Green%20Papers/Voluntary_Green_Paper.ashx?dl=true. Accessed 22 February 2010.

Conservative Party. (2022a). *Volunteer with us.* Landing page on the website. https://volunteer.conservatives.com/. Accessed 28 August 2022.

Covid-19 Mutual Aid UK. (2020a). *Frequently asked questions.* Page on the website of COVID-19 Mutual Aid UK. https://covidmutualaid.org/faq/. Accessed 27 June 2022.

Covid-19 Mutual Aid UK. (2022b). *Homepage.* Page on the website of Covid-19 Mutual Aid UK. https://covidmutualaid.org. Accessed 27 June 2022.

Cowman K. (2018). *What life was like as a suffragette organizer.* Blog on the website of the British Academy. https://www.thebritishacademy.ac.uk/blog/what-life-was-suffragette-organiser/. Accessed 27 August 2022.

Davis Smith, J. (1998). *The 1997 national survey of volunteering.* Institute for Volunteering Research.

Davis Smith, J. (2019). *100 years of NCVO and voluntary action: Idealists and realists.* Palgrave Macmillan.

Davis Smith, J., Rochester, C., & Hedley, R. (1995). *An introduction to the voluntary sector.* Routledge.

Delaney, S. (2014). *Making a big deal out of it, understanding volunteer management through applying psychological contract theory.* Paper on website of Voluntary Sector Studies Network, from VSSN Conference 2014 New researchers' sessions. http://www.vssn.org.uk/wp-content/uploads/2014/10/Abstract-and-paper-Shaun-Delaney.pdf. Accessed 28 August 2022.

Department for Communities and Local Government. (2010). *Volunteering for civic roles information for employers and employees*. Department for Communities and Local Government.

Department for Culture Media and Sport. (n.d.). *Enabling social action section A: A description of social action*. Department for Culture Media and Sport and New Economics Foundation. https://assets.publishing.service.gov.uk/government/uploads/system/uploads/attachment_data/file/591797/A_description_of_social_action.pdf. Accessed 26 June 2022.

Department for Digital, Culture, Media and Sport. (2020a). *Community life survey technical report 2019/20*. Department for Digital, Culture, Media and Sport.

Department for Digital, Culture, Media and Sport. (2020b). *3. Formal volunteering—Community life COVID-19 re-contact survey 2020*. Department for Digital, Culture, Media and Sport. https://www.gov.uk/government/statistics/community-life-covid-19-re-contact-survey-2020-main-report/3-formal-volunteering-community-life-recontact-survey-2020. Accessed 27 August 2022.

Department for Digital, Culture, Media and Sport. (2021). *Community Life Survey 2020/21*. Report on the webpages of the Department for Digital, Culture, Media and Sport. https://www.gov.uk/government/statistics/community-life-survey-202021. Accessed 27 August 2022.

Department for Digital, Culture, Media and Sport. (2022). *Government response to Danny Kruger MP's report: 'Levelling up our communities: Proposals for a new social covenant*. Page on the website of the Department for Digital, Culture, Media & Sport. https://www.gov.uk/government/publications/government-response-to-danny-kruger-mps-report-levelling-up-our-communities-proposals-for-a-new-social-covenant/government-response-to-danny-kruger-mps-report-levelling-up-our-communities-proposals-for-a-new-social-covenant. Accessed 27 August 2022.

Dewi, M. K., Manochin, M., & Belal, A. (2019). Marching with the volunteers: Their role and impact on beneficiary accountability in an Indonesian NGO. *Accounting, Auditing & Accountability Journal, 32*(4), 1117–1145. https://doi.org/10.1108/AAAJ-10-2016-2727

Do IT. (2022). *Amateur dramatics*. Page on the website of Do IT. https://doit.life/volunteering-opportunity/md/28778. Accessed 27 June 2022.

Donahue, K., McGarvey, A., Rooney, K., & Jochum, V. (2020). *Time well Spent: Diversity and volunteering research report December 2020*. National

Council for Voluntary Organisations. https://ncvo-app-wagtail-mediaa721
a567-uwkfinin077j.s3.amazonaws.com/documents/time_well_spent_divers
ity_and_volunteering_final.pdf. Accessed 28 August 2022]

Duke of Edinburgh's Award. (2021). *Annual report and financial state-
ments for the year ended 31 March 2021.* Duke of Edinburgh's
Award. https://www.dofe.org/wp-content/uploads/2022/01/JC0375_DofE-
Annual-Report_27_01_21.pdf. Accessed 26 June 2022.

Ellis Paine, A., Damm, C., Dean, J., Harris, C., & Macmillan, R. (2021).
Volunteering in community business: Meaning, practice and management.
Centre for Regional Economic and Social Research. https://www.shu.ac.
uk/-/media/home/research/cresr/reports/v/volunteering-in-community-bus
iness.pdf. Accessed 27 June 2022.

Field, A. (2016). *Why measuring impact is good for business.* Contribution on
Forbes Magazine website. https://www.forbes.com/sites/annefield/2016/
08/28/why-measuring-impact-is-good-for-business/?sh=10e8c67d7ddf.
Accessed 27 August 2022.

Greater London Volunteering. (2010). *Principles of volunteering, originally
agreed and endorsed by the London Stakeholders Volunteering Forum
and Member of GLV, 2009, Endorsed by the Members of GLV, 2010.*
Document available on the webpages of Greater London Volunteering. http://greaterlondonvolunteering.files.wordpress.com/2011/02/pri
nciplesofvolunteering.doc. Accessed 12 June 2022.

Green Party. (2022b). *Volunteer to get Greens elected.* Page on the website of the
Green Party. https://campaigns.greenparty.org.uk/get-involved/. Accessed 28
August 2022.

Greenpeace. (2022). *Join the political lobbying network.* Page on the website of
Greenpeace. https://www.greenpeace.org.uk/volunteering/join-the-political-
lobbying-network/. Accessed 12 June 2022.

Grotz, J. (1992). *Das Blindenwesen in der Volksrepublik China; Staatlicher
Anspruch und Realitat* (MA thesis). Marburg: Philipps-University.

Grotz, J. (2009). *The dignity and art of voluntary action—Voluntary action, a
human value or a commodity.* Paper delivered at ARNOVA's 38th Annual
Conference, November 19–22, 2009, Cleveland, Ohio, USA.

Grotz, J. (2010). *When volunteering goes wrong: Misconduct in volunteering.*
Paper delivered at 16th NCVO/VSSN Researching the Voluntary Sector
Conference, 6–7th September 2010, University of Leeds, UK.

Grotz, J. (2011). *Divisive, harmful and fatal: Less recognised impacts of volunteering.* Paper delivered at the NCVO/VSSN "Researching the Voluntary
Sector" Conference 7–8 September 2011, London.

Grotz J., Birt, L., Edwards, H., Locke M., & Poland F. (2021, February). Exploring disconnected discourses about patient and public involvement and volunteer involvement in English health and social care. *Health Expect, 24*(1), 8–18. https://doi.org/10.1111/hex.13162. Epub 2020 Dec 1. PMID: 33259704; PMCID: PMC7879540.

Grotz, J., Connolly, S., Woodard, R., & Parkinson, E. (2022). *Volunteering voices: A future vision for Hastings*. Institute for Volunteering Research.

Grotz, J., Ledgard, M., & Poland, F. (2020). *Patient and public involvement in health and social care: An introduction to theory and practice*. Imprint Springer Nature and Palgrave Macmillan.

Grotz, J., & Locke, M. (2022). *Volunteers and the law' versus 'volunteer rights,* Paper delivered at Voluntary Action History Society 7th International Conference, 13–15 July 2022, Liverpool.

Haldane, A. (2021). *The second invisible hand*. Local Trust Community Power Lecture. https://localtrust.org.uk/wp-content/uploads/2021/07/Andy-Haldane_Community-power-lecture_6-July.pdf. Accessed 28 August 2022.

Hardill, I., Grotz, J., & Crawford, L. (2022). *Mobilising voluntary action in the UK learning from the pandemic*. Policy Press.

Harris, B., Morris, A., Ascough, R. S., Chikoto, G. L., Elson, P. R., McLoughlin, J., Muukkonen, M., Pospíšilová, T., Roka, K., Smith, D. H., Soteri-Proctor, A., Tumanova, A. S., & Yu, P. J. (2016). History of associations and volunteering. In D. H. Smith, R. A. Stebbins, & J. Grotz (Eds.), *The Palgrave handbook of volunteering, civic participation, and nonprofit associations* (pp. 23–58). Palgrave Macmillan.

Higton, J., Archer, R., Merrett, D., Hansel, M., & Howe, P. (2021). *The community business market in 2020* (Research Institute Report No. 29). London: Power to Change.

Home Office. (2021). *Permission to work and volunteering for asylum seekers Version 10.0*. Home Office. https://assets.publishing.service.gov.uk/government/uploads/system/uploads/attachment_data/file/983283/permission-to-work-v10.0ext.pdf. Accessed 28 August 2022.

Howlett, S. (2010). Developing volunteer management as a profession. *Voluntary Sector Review, 1*(3), 355–360.

Hustinx, L., Cnaan, R. A., & Handy, F. (2010). Navigating theories of volunteering: A hybrid map for a complex phenomenon. *Journal for the Theory of Social Behaviour, 40*(4), 410–434. https://doi.org/10.1111/j.1468-5914.2010.00439.x

Illich, I. (1968). *Untitled talk delivered Saturday April 20 at St. Mary's Lake of the Woods Seminary in Niles (Chicago) Illinois, the talk is also referred to as 'to hell with good intentions'.* A text version of the speech was scanned from an original mimeograph distributed to Conference participants on the following day now available at The Conference on Interamerican Student Projects website. http://www.ciasp.ca/CIASPhistory/IllichCIASPspeech68.pdf. Accessed 26 June 2022.

Institute for Volunteering Research. (1998). *Issues in volunteer management—A report of a survey.* Institute for Volunteering Research.

Institute for Volunteering Research. (2004). *Volunteering for all: Exploring the link between volunteering and social exclusion.* Institute for Volunteering Research. https://www.bl.uk/collection-items/volunteering-for-all-exploring-the-link-between-volunteering-and-social-exclusion. Accessed 1 September 2022.

Institute for Volunteering Research. (2022). *Vision.* Page on the website of the Institute for Volunteering Research. https://www.uea.ac.uk/web/groups-and-centres/institute-for-volunteering-research/about-us. Accessed 27 August 2022.

Insulate Britain. (2022). *Help support the Insulate Britain Campaign.* Homepage of insulatebritain.com. http://insulatebritain.com. Accessed 27 June 2022.

Islamic Relief Worldwide. (2020). *Annual report and financial statements.* Islamic Relief Worldwide. https://www.islamic-relief.org.uk/wp-content/uploads/2021/08/IRW-AnnualReport2020-Signed.pdf. Accessed 26 June 2022.

Jackson, R., Locke, M., Hogg, E., & Lynch, R. (2019). *The complete volunteer management handbook* (4th ed.). Directory of Social Change.

Jewish Volunteering Network. (2019). *Annual review 2018–2019.* Jewish Volunteering Network. https://www.jvn.org.uk/files/?m=3255&s=1&l=1. Accessed 26 June 2022.

Johnson, B. (2021). *Prime Minister and head of the NHS call for volunteers to support National Booster Effort.* Press release on the website gov.uk. https://www.gov.uk/government/news/prime-ministeer-and-head-of-the-nhs-call-for-volunteers-to-support-national-booster-effort. Accessed 27 August 2022.

Kearney J. (2001). The values and basic principles of volunteering: Complacency or caution? *Voluntary Action, 3*(3), 63–86. Reprinted in Davis-Smith, J., & Locke, M. (Eds.). (2007). *Volunteering and the test of time: Essays for policy, organisation and research.* Institute for Volunteering Research.

Kropotkin, P. (1902). *Mutual aid: A factor of evolution.* Heineman.

Kruger, D. (2020). *Levelling up our communities: Proposals for a new social covenant A report for government by Danny Kruger MP.* A report posted on the website of Danny Kruger MP. https://www.dannykruger.org.uk/files/ 2020-09/Kruger%202.0%20Levelling%20Up%20Our%20Communities. pdf. Accessed 26 June 2022.

Labour Party. (2022c). *Volunteering FAQs*. Page on the website of The Labour Party. https://labour.org.uk/members/activist-area/budding-activists/ volunteering-faqs/. Accessed 28 August 2022.

Lampard, K., & Marsden, E. (2015). *Themes and lessons learnt from NHS investigations into matters relating to Jimmy Savile: Independent report for the Secretary of State for Health*. Report on the website assets.publishing.service.gov.uk. https://assets.publishing.service.gov.uk/ government/uploads/system/uploads/attachment_data/file/407209/KL_les sons_learned_report_FINAL.pdf. Accessed 28 May 2020.

Lawton, R., & Watt, W. (2019). *A Bit Rich: Why is volunteering biased towards higher socio-economic groups* (p. 12). Jump Projects.

Liberal Democrats. (2022). *Become a volunteer today*. Page on the website of the Liberal Democrats. https://www.libdems.org.uk/volunteer. Accessed 28 August 2022.

Local Government Information Unit. (2022). *Local government facts and figures: England*. Webpage on the website of the Local Government Information Unit. https://lgiu.org/local-government-facts-and-figures-england/#sec tion-4. Accessed 26 June 2022.

London School of Economic and Political Science Volunteer Centre. (2022). *About the LSE volunteer centre: Vision, mission and outcomes 2017–22*. Page on the Website of the London School of Economic and Political Science. https://info.lse.ac.uk/current-students/volunteer-centre/About-us. Accessed 26 June 2022.

Low, N., Butt, S., Ellis Paine, A., & Davis-Smith, J. (2007). *Helping out: A national survey of volunteering and charitable giving*. Cabinet Office.

Lukka, P., & Locke, M., with Soteri-Procter, A. (2003). *Faith and voluntary action: Community, values and resources*. Institute for Volunteering Research.

Madden, M., & Speed, E. (2017). Beware zombies and unicorns: Toward critical patient and public involvement in health research in a neoliberal context. *Frontiers in Sociology, 2*(7).

Magistrates Association. (2020). *Statistics published on diversity in the magistracy*. Page on the website of the Magistrates Association posted 29 September 2020. https://www.magistrates-association.org.uk/News-and-comments/statistics-published-on-diversity-in-the-magistracy. Accessed 27 June 2022.

Mason, R. (2014). *Charities should stick to knitting and keep out of politics, says MP*. The Guardian News Webpages 3 September 2014. https://www.theguardian.com/society/2014/sep/03/charities-knitting-politics-brook-newmark. Accessed 25 June 2022.

May, C. (2018). *DUCK expeditions are a load of quack*. Comments on webpages of student publication Palatinate posted 2 April 2018. https://www.palatinate.org.uk/duck-expeditions-are-a-load-of-quack/. Accessed 25 June 2022.

McCabe, A., Wilson, M., Macmillan, R., & Ellis Paine, A. (2021). *Now they see us: Communities responding to COVID-19*. Report on the website of the Local Trust. https://localtrust.org.uk/wp-content/uploads/2021/07/Now-they-see-us.pdf. Accessed 25 June 2022.

McCord, J. (2003). Cures that harm: Unanticipated outcomes of crime prevention programs. *Annals of the American Academy of Political and Social Science, 587*, 16–30.

McGarvey, A., Jochum, V., & Chan, O. (2019a). *Time well spent: Employer-supported volunteering* (Research Report). London: National Council for Voluntary Organisations. https://www.befriending.co.uk/resources/24751-time-well-spent-employer-supported-volunteering. Accessed 27 August 2022.

McGarvey, A., Jochum, V., Chan, O., Delaney, S., Young, R., & Gillies, C. (2020). *Time well spent: Volunteering in the public sector* (Research Report). London: National Council for Voluntary Organisations. https://www.befriending.co.uk/r/24836-time-well-spent-volunteering-in-the-public-sector. Accessed 27 August 2022.

McGarvey, A., Jochum, V., Davies, J., Dobbs, J., & Hornung, L. (2019b). *Time well spent: A national survey on the volunteer experience*. NCVO.

Meakin, B., & Grotz, J. (2020). *Throwing away the rulebook: Five things you should consider when planning interactive online events, to make them more inclusive*. Blog on the webpages of the Applied Research Collaboration East of England. https://arc-eoe.nihr.ac.uk/node/271. Accessed 27 August 2022.

Miliband, E. (2011). *Responsibility in the 21st century*. Transcript of speech on website of politics.co.uk. https://www.politics.co.uk/comment-analysis/2011/06/13/ed-miliband-responsibility-speech-in-full/. Accessed 25 June 2022.

Mohan, J., & Bulloch, S. L. (2012). *The idea of a 'civic core': What are the overlaps between charitable giving, volunteering, and civic participation in England and Wales?* (Third Sector Research Centre Working Paper

73). https://www.birmingham.ac.uk/Documents/college-social-sciences/social-policy/tsrc/working-papers/working-paper-73.pdf. Accessed 27 August 2022.

Mulgan, G. (n.d.). *Measuring our impact: The measurement of innovation impact is rarely straightforward but it's essential to try and track what is being achieved*. Contribution on webpages of NESTA. https://www.nesta.org.uk/feature/measuring-our-impact/?gclid=EAIaIQobChMIgZyPy7bG-QIVY2HmCh1SSAJvEAAYASAAEgKS2_D_BwE. Accessed 27 August 2022.

Murray, P., Shea, J., & Hoare, G. (2017). *Charities taking charge: transforming to face a changing world*. New Philanthropy Capital. https://www.thinknpc.org/resource-hub/charities-taking-charge/. Accessed 27 August 2022.

National Citizen Service Trust. (2022). *About NCS Trust*. Page on the website of the National Citizen Service Trust. https://wearencs.com/about-ncs-trust. Accessed 28 August 2022.

National Council for Voluntary Organisations. (n.d.). *If volunteering goes wrong*. Page on the website of the National Council for Voluntary Organisations. https://www.ncvo.org.uk/get-involved/volunteering/if-volunteering-goes-wrong/. Accessed 27 August 2022.

National Council for Voluntary Organisations. (2014a). *Report of the inquiry into charity senior executive pay*. National Council for Voluntary Organisations. https://www.ncvo.org.uk/images/news/Executive-Pay-Report.pdf. Accessed 27 June 2022.

National Council for Voluntary Organisations. (2014b). *Final report of the call to action progress group following the volunteer rights inquiry*. National Council for Voluntary Organisations. http://blogs.ncvo.org.uk/wp-content/uploads/mike-locke/call-to-action-progress-group-volunteer-rights-inquiry-report.pdf. Accessed 25 June 2022.

National Council for Voluntary Organisations. (2018). *Impactful Volunteering, understanding the impact of volunteering on volunteers*. Research briefing on National Council for Voluntary Organisations webpages. https://www.ncvo.org.uk/images/documents/policy_and_research/Impactful-volunteering-understanding-the-impact-of-volunteering-on-volunteers.pdf. Accessed 25 June 2022.

National Council for Voluntary Organisations. (2020). *Time well spent: Volunteering in the public sector, research report*. National Council for Voluntary Organisations. https://www.befriending.co.uk/r/24836-time-well-spent-volunteering-in-the-public-sector. Accessed 27 June 2022.

National Council for Voluntary Organisations. (2021). *UK Civil Society Almanac 2021: Data trends insights*. Executive summary on webpages of

National Council for Voluntary Organisations. https://www.ncvo.org.uk/news-and-insights/news-index/uk-civil-society-almanac-2021/. Accessed 27 August 2022.

National Trust. (2021). *Annual report 2020/21.* National Trust. https://nt.global.ssl.fastly.net/documents/annual-report-202021.pdf. Accessed 27 June 2022.

Naylor, C., Mundle, C., Weaks, L., & Buck, D. (2013). *Volunteering in health and care: Securing a sustainable future.* Kings Fund. https://www.kingsfund.org.uk/sites/default/files/field/field_publication_file/volunteering-in-health-and-social-care-kingsfund-mar13.pdf. Accessed 26 June 2022.

New Local. (2022). *About.* Page in the website of New Local. www.newlocal.org.uk/about/. Accessed 29 August 2022.

NewStatesman Archive. (2021). *From the NS archive: Mr Chamberlain's fiasco 7 April 1917: A call for volunteers, but volunteering for what?* https://www.newstatesman.com/2021/05/ns-archive-mr-chamberlain-s-fiasco. Accessed 27 August 2022. The authors are grateful to Dr Sandy MacDonald, University of Northampton for pointing out this report for the evidence collection of the project https://www.mvain4.uk

NHS England. (2017). *Recruiting and managing volunteers in NHS providers: A practical guide.* NHS England. https://www.england.nhs.uk/wp-content/uploads/2017/10/recruiting-managing-volunteers-nhs-providers-practical-guide.pdf. Accessed 4 August 2022.

NHS England. (2019). *The NHS long term plan.* NHS England. https://www.longtermplan.nhs.uk/wp-content/uploads/2019/08/nhs-long-term-plan-version-1.2.pdf. Accessed 27 August 2022.

Ockenden, N. (Ed.). (2007). *Volunteering works: Volunteering and social policy.* Institute for Volunteering Research and Volunteering England.

Ockenden, N., & Hutin, M. (2008). *Volunteering to lead: A study of leadership in small volunteer led groups IVR 2008* (p. 35). Institute for Volunteering Research.

O'Hagan, M. (2001). *Stories from the edge.* Volunteer Development Agency, Northern Ireland. https://www.yumpu.com/en/document/read/52071572/stories-from-the-edge-volunteer-now. Accessed 27 August 2022.

Parentkind. (2021). *Report and accounts for the year ended 31 December 2020.* Parentkind.

Power, A., & Benton, E. (2021). *Where next for Britain's 4,300 mutual aid groups?* Blog on the website of LSE. https://blogs.lse.ac.uk/covid19/2021/05/06/where-next-for-britains-4300-mutual-aid-groups/. Accessed 27 August 2022.

Preston, J., & Firth, R. (2020). *Coronavirus, class and mutual aid in the United Kingdom.* Palgrave Macmillan.

Prince's Trust Group. (2021). *Annual report and accounts 2020/21.* Prince's Trust Group. https://www.princes-trust.org.uk/about-the-trust/research-policies-reports/annual-report. Accessed 28 June 2022.

Putnam, R. D. (2000). *Bowling alone, the collapse and revival of American community.* Simon and Schuster Paperbacks.

Ricketts, A. (2022). *Re-establishing volunteer and giving levels will require 'active and co-ordinated efforts', think tank warns.* Contribution on the website of ThirdSector. https://www.thirdsector.co.uk/re-establishing-volunteer-giving-levels-will-require-active-co-ordinated-efforts-think-tank-warns/management/article/1787403. Accessed 29 May 2022.

Robinson, D. (2020). *The moment we noticed: The relationships observatory and our learning from 100 days of lockdown.* Relationships Project. https://relationshipsproject.org/content/uploads/2020/07/The-Moment-We-Noticed_RelationshipsProject_202.pdf. Accessed 27 August 2022.

Rochester, C. (1999). One size does not fit all: Four models of involving volunteers in small voluntary organisations. *Voluntary Action, 1*(2), 7–20.

Rochester, C. (2013). *Rediscovering voluntary action.* Palgrave Macmillan.

Rochester, C., Ellis Paine, A., Howlett, S., with Zimmeck, M. (2010). *Volunteering and society in the 21st century.* Palgrave Macmillan.

Rosenberg, T. (2018). *The business of voluntourism: Do western do-gooders actually do harm?* Contribution on the Guardian website. https://www.theguardian.com/news/2018/sep/13/the-business-of-voluntourism-do-western-do-gooders-actually-do-harm. Accessed 27 August 2022.

Ross, M. W., Greenfield, S. A., & Bennett, L. (1999). Predictors of dropout and burnout in AIDS volunteers: A longitudinal study. *AIDS Care, 11*(6), 723–731.

Rotary. (2022). *About Rotary.* Page on Rotary Website. https://www.rotary.org/en/get-involved/rotary-clubs. Accessed 27 June 2022a.

Royal National Lifeboat Institution. (2020). *RNLI annual report and accounts 2020: A year like no other.* Royal National Lifeboat Institution. https://rnli.org/about-us/how-the-rnli-is-run/annual-report-and-accounts. Accessed 26 June 2022.

Royal Society for the Protection of Birds. (2022). *Our history.* Page on the website of the Royal Society for the Protection of Birds. https://www.rspb.org.uk/about-the-rspb/about-us/our-history/. Accessed 28 June 2022.

Scottish Government. (2019). *Volunteering for all: Our national framework*. Scottish Government. https://www.gov.scot/publications/volunteering-national-framework/. Accessed 27 June 2022.

Scottish Government. (2022). *Scotland's volunteering action plan*. Scottish Government. https://www.gov.scot/publications/scotlands-volunteering-action-plan/. Accessed 26 July 2022.

Slawson, N. (2016). *The public services you didn't know were run by charities*. News on The Guardian webpages published 20 May 2016. https://www.theguardian.com/voluntary-sector-network/2016/may/20/10-public-services-run-charities. Accessed 27 June 2022.

Smith, D. H. (2000). *Grassroots associations*. Sage.

Smith, D. H. (2019). *A review of deviant nonprofit groups: Seeking method in their alleged 'madness-treason-immorality'*. Brill.

Smith, D. H., Stebbins, R. A., & Grotz, J. (Eds.). (2016). *The Palgrave handbook of volunteering, civic participation, and nonprofit associations*. Palgrave Macmillan.

Smith, K., & Holmes, K. (2009). Researching volunteers in tourism: Going beyond. *Annals of Leisure Research, 12*(3/4), 403–420.

Sport England. (2016). *Volunteering in an active nation*. Sport England. https://sportengland-production-files.s3.eu-west-2.amazonaws.com/s3fs-public/2020-01/volunteering-in-an-active-nation-final.pdf?VersionId=LU3cqHb9FZvVWi3rye.b.HNIe5UM9wOX. Accessed 26 June 2022.

St John Ambulance. (2021). *Humanity in crisis: Annual report and accounts for the year ended 31 December 2020*. St John Ambulance. https://www.sja.org.uk/globalassets/documents/annual-reports-and-accounts/st-john-ambulance-annual-report-2020_web.pdf. Accessed 26 June 2022.

Stebbins, R., & Graham, M. (Eds.). (2004). *Volunteering as leisure/leisure as volunteering: An International Assessment*. CABI Publishing.

Stoker, J. (2008). *Report of a review by John Stoker of York Citizens Advice Bureau*. Citizens Advice. http://www.citizensadvice.org.uk/pdf_review_yorkcab_report.pdf. Accessed 31 August 2010.

Stuart, J., Kamerāde, D., Connolly, S., Ellis Paine, A., Nichols, G., & Grotz, J. (2020). *The impacts of volunteering on the subjective wellbeing of volunteers: A rapid evidence assessment*. London: What Works Centre for Wellbeing and Spirit of 2012. https://whatworkswellbeing.org/wp-content/uploads/2020/10/Volunteer-wellbeing-technical-report-Oct2020-a.pdf. Accessed 31 May 2022.

Surfers Against Sewage. (2022). *Organise your million mile clean.* Page on the website of Surfers Against Sewage. https://www.sas.org.uk/our-work/beach-cleans/organise-beach-clean. Accessed 26 June 2022.

Syed, M. (2019). *Rebel ideas: The power of diverse thinking.* John Murray.

Taylor, P., Nichols, G., Holmes, K., James, M., Gratton, C., Garrett, R., Kokolakakis, T., Mulder, C., & King, L. (2003). *Sports volunteering in England 2002: A report for Sports England.* Leisure Industries Research Centre. https://sportengland-production-files.s3.eu-west-2.amazonaws.com/s3fs-public/valuing-volunteering-in-sport-in-england-final-report.pdf. Accessed 26 June 2022.

Teasdale, S. (2008a). *In good health: Assessing the impact of volunteering in the NHS.* Volunteering England.

Teasdale, S. (2008b). *Health check: A practical guide to assessing the impact of volunteering in the NHS.* Volunteering England.

Thoits, P. A., & Hewitt, L. N. (2001). Volunteer work and well-being. *Journal of Health and Social Behavior, 42*(2), 115–131.

Thomas, B. (2006). Assessing the impact of volunteering in a London borough. *Voluntary Action, 8*(1), 92–103.

Thomas, T. (2022). *Insulate Britain protesters praised by judge who fined them.* News on The Guardian webpages published 13 April 2022. https://www.theguardian.com/environment/2022/apr/13/insulate-britain-protesters-praised-by-judge-who-fined-them. Accessed 28 June 2022.

Tiratelli, L., & Kaye, K. (2020). *Communities vs. coronavirus: The rise of mutual aid.* New Local. https://www.newlocal.org.uk/wp-content/uploads/2020/12/Communities-vs-Coronavirus_New-Local.pdf. Accessed 27 August 2022.

Trades Union Congress. (2009). *A charter for strengthening relations between paid staff and volunteers.* A page on the website of the Trades Union Congress. https://www.tuc.org.uk/research-analysis/reports/charter-strengthening-relations-between-paid-staff-and-volunteers. Accessed 27 August 2022.

Tseloni, A., & Tura, F. (2019). *Neighbourhood watch membership: Trends, obstacles, members' and potential members' profiles executive summary.* Nottingham Trent University. https://www.ourwatch.org.uk/sites/default/files/documents/2020-01/Neighbourhood%20Watch%20Membership%20exetutive%20summary.pdf. Accessed 27 June 2022.

Twigg, J., & Mosel, I. (2017). Emergent groups and spontaneous volunteers in urban disaster response. *Environment and Urbanization, 29*(2), 443–458.

https://doi.org/10.1177/0956247817721413 https://journals.sagepub.com/doi/full/10.1177/0956247817721413. Accessed 28 June 2022.

Unison. (2018a). *Crossing the line, police support volunteers: Rising numbers and mission creep*. Unison. https://www.unison.org.uk/content/uploads/2019/01/Report_on_Police_upport-Volunteers_2018a.pdf. Accessed 12 June 2022.

Unison. (2018b). *Volunteers taking on police roles as cuts continue to bite*. Post on the Unison webpages, 7 December 2018. https://www.unison.org.uk/news/press-release/2018/12/volunteers-taking-police-roles-cuts-continue-bite/. Accessed 12 June 2022.

Unison. (n.d.). *Volunteers*. Guidance on the website of Unison. https://www.unison.org.uk/content/uploads/2016/01/Volunteers.pdf. Accessed 5 August 2022.

United Nations General Assembly. (2001a). *UNGA Resolution 56/38: Recommendations on support for volunteering*. Page on website of UN Volunteers. https://www.unv.org/publications/unga-resolution-5638-recommendations-support-volunteering. Accessed 28 June 2022.

United Nations General Assembly. (2001b). *Support for volunteering: Report of the secretary-general*. Page on the website of the United Nations. https://www.un.org/webcast/events/iyv/a56288.pdf. Accessed 27 August 2022.

United Nations Volunteers (UNV) Programme. (2021). *2022 state of the world's volunteerism report. Building equal and inclusive societies*. United Nations Volunteers (UNV) programme.

Vision for Volunteering. (2020). *How does volunteering need to adapt by 2032?* Landing page on the website of the Vision for Volunteering. https://www.visionforvolunteering.org.uk. Accessed 27 August 2022.

Volans, I. (2010). *Die Turnhalle: Britains first gymnasium*. Page on the website SportingLandmarks.co.uk. https://sportinglandmarks.co.uk/die-turnhalle-britains-first-gymnasium/. Accessed 27 August 2022.

Volunteering England. (2008). *Volunteering England information sheet: Definitions of volunteering*. Volunteering England. http://www.volunteering.org.uk/NR/rdonlyres/4C135BDF-E1E2-43D4-8FD8-DB16AE4536AA/0/DefinitionsofVolunteeringVE08.pdf. Accessed 22 February 2010.

Volunteering England. (2009). *Volunteering England information sheet: If things go wrong*. Volunteering England. http://www.volunteering.org.uk/NR/rdonlyres/BD1C333F-18EF-4FA3-BD66-90780982DF51/0/ISIfThingsGoWrongVE09.pdf. Accessed 31 August 2010.

Volunteering England. (2010). *Volunteer rights inquiry: Interim report*. Volunteering England.

Volunteering England. (2011). *The practical guide to employer supported volunteering for employers*. Volunteering England.

Volunteer Now. (2022). *Working with volunteers—Problem solving procedures*. Page on the website of Volunteer Now. https://www.volunteernow.co.uk/app/uploads/2022/05/Problem-Solving-Procedures-1.pdf. Accessed 27 August 2022.

Volunteer Rights Inquiry. (2010). *Interim report*. Volunteering England. http://www.volunteering.org.uk/NR/rdonlyres/742EBA26-A6CB-4531-BBBB-7C2A35CCE5D5/0/VE_volunteering_inquiry_FIN_web.pdf. Accessed 31 August 2010.

Ward, L. (2017). *Charities are asking interns to work 252 hours unpaid. That's a scandal*. News on The Guardian webpages published 30 November 2017. https://www.theguardian.com/voluntary-sector-network/2017/nov/30/charities-interns-unpaid-work-scandal-volunteering-experience. Accessed 16 June 2022.

We are right here. (2022). *New research: Covid mutual aid groups are here to stay*. Page on the website of 'We are right here: The Campaign for Community Power'. https://www.right-here.org/new-research-covid-mutual-aid-groups-are-here-to-stay/. Accessed 27 August 2022.

Weiss, C. H. (1972). *Evaluation research: Methods for assessing program effectiveness*. Prentice Hall.

Wilkinson, N., & Long, R. (2019). *School governance: Briefing paper number 08072, 17 December 2019*. House of Commons Library. https://researchbriefings.files.parliament.uk/documents/CBP-8072/CBP-8072.pdf. Accessed 26 June 2022.

Wilson, J. (2000). Volunteering. *Annual Review of Sociology, 26*, 215–240.

Wolch, J. (1990). *The shadow state: Government and voluntary sector in transition*. The Foundation Centre.

Wolfenden Committee. (1978). *The future of voluntary organisations*. Croom Helm.

Women's Institutes of England, Wales, Jersey, Guernsey and the Isle of Man. (2021). *Report and financial statements for the year ended 30 September 2021*. Women's Institutes of England, Wales, Jersey, Guernsey and the Isle of Man. https://www.thewi.org.uk/__data/assets/pdf_file/0008/569681/NFWI-Signed-Trustees-Annual-Return-for-September-2021.pdf. Accessed 27 June 2022.

Workers' Educational Association. (2022). *About us*. Webpages of the https://www.wea.org.uk/. https://www.wea.org.uk/about-us. Accessed 26 June 2022.

Wyper, H. (2001). *The outlook for branch/group networks of national charities: What can be learnt from a survey of relevant organisations?* [Dissertation]. Centre for Voluntary Sector and Not-for-Profit Management City University Business School.

Young, N. M. (2012). *Volunteer centre network 'will fragment' under council cuts.* Page on Civil Society News website. https://www.civilsociety.co.uk/news/volunteer-centre-network--will-fragment--under-council-cuts.html. Accessed 27 August 2022.

Youth Hostel Association. (2022). *Complete your award with us DofE: Can we count you in?* Pages on https://volunteer.yha.org.uk/. https://volunteer.yha.org.uk/index-classic. Accessed 26 June 2022.

Zimmeck, M. (2010). Government and volunteering: Towards a history of policy and practice. In C. Rochester, E. P. Angela, & S. Howlett, with M. Zimmeck (Eds.), *Volunteering and society in the 21st century* (pp. 84–102). Palgrave Macmillan.

Index

© The Author(s), under exclusive license to Springer Nature Switzerland AG 2022
J. Grotz and R. Leonard, *Volunteer Involvement*,
https://doi.org/10.1007/978-3-031-19221-0

Printed in the United States
by Baker & Taylor Publisher Services